The Urbana Free Library

To renew: call **217-367-4057**
or go to **urbanafreelibrary.org**
and select **My Account**

EMBRACE

For Mathew, Oliver, Cruz, Mikaela,
Bettyanne, Geoffrey, Justine, Jason,
Ben, Charlotte, Lily and Aunty Ronda...
my everything.

EMBRACE

MY STORY FROM BODY LOATHER
TO BODY LOVER

Taryn Brumfitt

NEW
HOLLAND

First published in 2015 by New Holland Publishers Pty Ltd
London · Sydney · Auckland

The Chandlery, Unit 9, 50 Westminster Bridge Road, London SE1 7QY, United Kingdom
1/66 Gibbes Street, Chatswood, NSW 2067, Australia
218 Lake Road, Northcote, Auckland 0627, New Zealand

www.newhollandpublishers.com

A record of this book is held at the British Library and the National Library
of Australia.

ISBN: 978 1 74257 618 3

Managing Director: Fiona Schultz
Publisher: Diane Ward
Project Editor: Joanne Rippin
Designer: Thomas Casey
Production Director: Olga Dementiev
Photographs: Andre Agnew, Kate Ellis, Benjamin Liew, Karen Pfieffer, David Solm
Printer: Toppan Leefung Printing Ltd

10 9 8 7 6 5 4 3 2 1

Keep up with New Holland Publishers on Facebook
www.facebook.com/NewHollandPublishers

CONTENTS

FOREWORD

By Ricki Lake

AS SOMEONE WHO HAS STRUGGLED WITH MY BODY IMAGE over the years, and been watched and judged by the media while I do so, it is inspiring to see someone like Taryn take a stand against the way society pressurises women to conform to a certain shape.

From time to time I have wished I'd been born in a different body and didn't have to struggle with my weight, or the way that I look hadn't had such a negative effect on my self-confidence, but let's face it, my big break wouldn't have happened if I'd been a size 4 at that point. So I guess it's important to be happy with what you've got; we're all unique and special in our own way and there is beauty in all of it.

I've had a very complex love/hate relationship with my body, and this was exacerbated when director John Waters chose me to be the 'fat girl' in his movie, *Hairspray*. I felt like I was a walking contradiction; on the one hand I became a star and everybody loved the character of this adorable chubby girl, and yet deep down inside I was still struggling to find myself, and be comfortable in my own skin. I feel like much of my adult life has been spent dealing with this inner conflict, trying to find my natural body; I've been 120 pounds and I've been 260 pounds, from size 4 to 24.

I would like women in the next generation to struggle less than I have, it would be great if we started showing real women in magazines and on TV, and went back to appreciating women of all shapes and sizes. I have sons, I don't have daughters, but even with my sons it pains me to think about what I'm passing onto them when they hear me complain about my weight when we're together; it's such an unhealthy, almost involuntary habit. We're so messed up about what we put into our bodies and how we take care of ourselves, and facing it is a conversation that needs to be had.

This is why I love what Taryn is doing with her book and her documentary. Like many other women in this image-conscious modern world, she has struggled to escape from the effects of hating her own body. And now she's encouraging women to stop obsessing about the size of their boobs or belly and just go out, do stuff and enjoy life. Eat healthily, fuel your body so it has lots of energy, use natural products rather than chemicals and try your best to make sure you don't pass on your own body neuroses to the next generation.

It sounds simple, but of course it isn't, it's a process. I wish I could be one of those women that could just get over it, it's a real struggle. But I resent the fact that so many days of my life have been lost to being dissatisfied with my body. And if we agree that we've had enough, and we're going to take back the power we've allowed the media to have over our self-image, maybe that will be a start. I think projects like Taryn's Body Image Movement are the way to make this happen; it needs to start from the ground up, not the other way around.

Reading Taryn's book is like making a new best friend. Her caring personality shines through everything she writes about, whether it's her hilarious physical embarrassments and humiliations, which we'll all recognise, or her passionate attacks against the diet industry that she feels continually rips us off. I thoroughly recommend this book to all women, of every shape and size, and I suggest those women then pass it on to their daughters, nieces, goddaughters... and sons!

Ricki Lake 2014

CHAPTER ONE

Bright lights and porno shoes

'DO I HAVE A CAMEL TOE? Oh my God! Hi, I'm Taryn, do I have a camel toe?' Fuck, they are about to call my name and I think I've wedged my briefs up too far. I've always been a self-confessed Harry high pants, and generally I can get away with it by throwing a big sloppy sweater over the top. On this occasion there is nowhere for this bad boy camel toe to hide. Finally I find a girl that uses words to respond to my question, not just the doe-eyed confused look I got from the first two. 'Um, I can't see, it's a bit dark.' Helpful.

The next thing I hear is, 'Please welcome Taryn Brumfitt onto the stage.' That's me. Madonna is playing so it is definitely meant to be me. I've got this. Oh my, these lights are so bright. I can see my dad's silver fox hair in the audience. 'Hi Dad' (nervous giggle) in my head. The stage is bright, the audience is dark and yet I can make out a lot of faces. There are over seven hundred people watching me on stage, strutting in a teeny tiny sparkling silver bikini and porno shoes. A fitness model, competing with twenty other girls in a bodybuilding competition for one of Australia's most respected bodybuilding federations.

How did I end up here? What was I thinking? This is hilarious! I wish the audience knew my story. I wonder how inappropriate it would be to ask the dude with the microphone for a bit of airtime? Probably very inappropriate – okay just smile then.

Inside my head I am laughing. I am laughing so hard that it almost drowns out the feeling of sheer terror from a) being on a stage in front of a bunch of people, and b) being on a stage in front of a bunch of people wearing a bikini! I strut across the stage and all I can think is, 'Please don't fall over on a stage in front of an audience, in a bikini, wearing porno shoes.' My legs are trembling and my breathing is shallow. I make it to the other side of the stage. Take that, judges, with your hypercritical ogling eyes piercing through to my soul. I didn't fall over, surely I deserve a little wink or a smile for that. Not a chance. Then I remember; I'm not here to be measured on how well I can walk in these ridiculously ugly shoes, neither is my personality or talent being assessed, it is my body that is being judged. As I move closer to the MC the urge to grab the microphone gets stronger, inside my head I believe that in this moment I could deliver a speech on body love and acceptance that would rival any Anthony Robbins motivational rant. Taryn, calm the fuck down, resist the microphone, you are not here to be listened to, you are here to be looked at. Ouch, a part of the feminist inside me crumbles.

I take a moment to remind myself of the reasons I am here. This was a social experiment that started fifteen weeks ago when I uttered the words, 'I wonder what it feels like to have the perfect body?' to my personal trainer, Ruth.

Unsurprisingly I had met Ruth at the gym, she took a boxing class on Saturdays and she was merciless. I loved her spirit and her strength, she meant business, and for me, who likes to work hard and channel my inner Demi Moore from the movie *G.I Jane*, she was the perfect fit.

Boxing has always been my choice of exercise. At my work experience from school I chose to go to the gym and learn how to box, because I thought at the tender age of fifteen that following in the footsteps of Rocky Balboa was a really good idea. I remember the school counsellor attempting to guide me in another direction and I clearly remember asking him why he didn't think being a competitive athlete was an ambitious enough goal. I also remember asking him whether his resistance to my choice of 'work experience' was because I was a girl. Of course it wasn't, I was just being an annoying smart ass and pushing the boundaries, because that's just what you do when you're a fifteen-year-old whippersnapper who eats raw eggs for breakfast.

The training schedule Ruth planned out was relentless. I had exactly fifteen weeks from the time I had committed to training until the day I stepped on stage. I started training the day after Australia Day. I remember it well because I spent the entire training session fighting back the urge to throw up. As Australia Day was going to be my last day of food and alcohol freedom for nearly four months, I did what any other good Australian would do – I went to the Australia Day Cricket Test and gave it a really good nudge.

At test cricket matches in Australia you don't really watch too much of the game. You do a lot of drinking, have childish water fights, wear random men's watermelon helmets and sing, 'Aussie Aussie Aussie Oi Oi Oi,' a lot. It's a place where you feed your inner bogan, unless of course you are in the members section, in which case you'll be knocking back chilled Sauvignon Blanc, chowing down on fancy canapés and pretending to be more important than you actually are. I hear that chicken soup is good for the soul, I say a day at the cricket is even better. One thing's for sure, deciding to spend a day at the cricket before a Day One 'Let's set the tone' training session is an epic fail at best.

So I (just) got through Day One of training and at the time I thought it was a tough session. Little did I know that the next one hundred sessions would be just as hard, if not harder. I was up at 5.30am, six days a week, and I ran, lifted weights, cycled, squat jumped, punched, kicked, sweated and on occasions pushed myself so hard that I would actually throw up. Halfway through my training schedule, I went from one training session a day to two. Cardio to begin the day on an empty stomach, then weights later in the evening, somewhere between kids dinner at 5pm and bedtime at 7pm. (Kids' bedtime that is, although I was so smashed most nights that I probably could've put myself to bed at the same time.)

I had to work so hard for my bikini body because I had such a short training time. Most competing girls would train for at least 9–12 months prior to the competition date. Hard and fast was my motto, and I was told constantly by Ruth to give it all I had and leave nothing in the tank, because I had tough competition. The reality was, I never felt like I was competing against the other girls, all I aimed for was to blend in and not stick out like a sore thumb.

There was one training session that I will never forget. It was the week of the competition and I had been advised to indulge in a little carb-loading. Increasing carbohydrate intake is a strategy mostly used by endurance athletes to maximise the storage of glycogen (energy) in the muscles. Basically, the purpose of carb-loading for the bodybuilding competition was to give my muscles a larger appearance as well as help tighten up the loose skin around my tummy. First though I had to become carb-free; for three days I ate only chicken and broccoli and then on the Thursday I headed to the gym and worked out for nearly four hours. The idea was to deplete the muscles of any glycogen and then build it up over the 48 hours before my big stage debut.

Ruth arrived when I had been on the treadmill for two hours and I was dripping with sweat and exhausted. I'd run nearly a half marathon and I felt like there was nothing in the tank, but of course there was, and she got it out of me. After a quick clothes change we went into the weights room for a gruelling circuit that lasted another two hours. At the end I couldn't move, I wasn't broken or in tears like Demi Moore, but I certainly was unable to string a proper sentence together or walk all that well.

Physical training complete I now had to get beautified. For someone who doesn't wear makeup very often, and doesn't use chemicals (on skin or in food) I was in for a real treat. Hair, makeup, spray tan, nails, more spray tan and a lot of hair removing. It honestly felt like I was getting married again. The spray tanning sessions were interesting, thank God the beautician was an adorable and friendly woman, because standing butt naked while someone is kneeling in front of you spraying your inner thigh is not for the faint hearted! When I got home after my tan my husband Mat didn't even recognise me, and when he did, he just laughed, in fact he was in hysterics. I did look really bizarre, my tic tac shaped teeth shining brightly against my mahogany-coloured skin.

Arriving backstage on the evening of the competition, I was incredibly nervous. Lots of the girls obviously knew each other and seemed to belong to a group, and I noticed immediately that I was the most senior, by a long way. These girls were really young! I reckon I had about ten years on the oldest of them.

Backstage there was a big open room where guys and girls were happily changing, applying oils and preening, and at the back there was a smaller room. I headed straight there, I was far too nervous to get my kit off and get ready in front of one hundred strangers. When I opened the door of this small room, there were already about a dozen girls there, I declared my name, gave them a detailed update about how I was feeling, dumped my bag down and started to get my clothes off. When I looked up from pulling my trackies down, I noticed they were all staring back at me, and their glares weren't friendly. Someone whom I later found out was the 'coach' of the girls, said to me in THE most patronising voice, 'This is our private room where we get ready, and we like to get ready alone.' I felt a flutter in the pit of my stomach, similar to the one I regularly felt at high school when I got bullied (another story for another chapter). My heart sank, I was really embarrassed and I dealt with it the way I know best, a little humour and too much talking. Seriously, when shit hits the fan and I'm around you can be guaranteed that I will get verbal diarrhoea. 'Oh ladies, how awkward is this?!' (Insert sounds of crickets.) 'First competition, don't know too many people, and here I am, in the wrong place. With you.' (Insert nervous laugh.) 'Well, I am sure there is a spot through that door just for me, myself and I, and I'm going to go find it, right...' (They are still staring.) '... Now.' Sheesh, these girls are a tough crowd, I note that my tracksuit pants are still around my ankles (why did I wear runners and not thongs like everyone else?). I pull up my pants, grab my bags and get the truck out of there.

It is busy everywhere, so I set up my station in the middle of a walkway. I look around, there are women doing exercises with stretchy bands, hairspray being sprayed, gloss being applied – I'm not in Kansas anymore Toto.

I go to the toilets, put my bikini on and put my singlet back on over the top. Ruth says, 'Why are you wearing that singlet?' To which I reply, 'I don't want anyone to see me in my bikini.' Ruth gives me the most perplexed look, 'Taryn, you are about to go on stage in front of hundreds of people, get your singlet off.' I feel completely exposed, and it is in that moment that the enormity of what I was about to do hits home. I feel a wave of sickness come over me, but before I can work myself up into a real state, it is time to head up the stairs and wait backstage for my name to be called. So I hoick my bikini bottoms up as high as possible, and off I go.

So here I am on stage, outwardly smiling but internally laughing at the outrageous notion that I, Taryn Brumfitt, am on a stage in a bikini and porno shoes, possibly with a camel toe (not that we will ever know). How could it possibly be that such a short time ago I was on the bathroom floor, crying my eyes out and loathing every inch of my body. How did I get here? Well, it's a long story and it started seven years ago, sitting in a commode chair in a hospital...

CHAPTER TWO

The commode chair

'OH DEAR GOD, HERE COMES ANOTHER ONE,' I scream, doubled over the kitchen bench. I look up to see eight tradesmen staring at me through the glass wall of the extension we were building at the back of the house, and as my eyes meet theirs they immediately look away and go back to hammering, drilling and sanding. The house renovation was supposed to be finished by the time the baby arrived, but we were running weeks over schedule.

Once the contraction had finished I took the opportunity to head outside and engage in some friendly banter with the lads, cracking predictable and completely unfunny jokes about getting it done faster because the baby is on its way. Doubling over once more I realised it wasn't the time for jokes; it was time to get to the hospital.

Arriving at the hospital I enthusiastically hand over my birth plan to the midwife, it's imperative that she and her team understand my very well-thought out ideas of how I want the day to progress; how I want to be communicated with throughout the labour. Only a few months before, Mat and I had spent a considerable amount of money on a hypnobirthing weekend workshop, and by God were we going to get our money's worth, using all of our new skills to ensure the birth was quiet, calm and tranquil.

Fast forward eight hours and all thoughts of tranquility, serenity and harmony had been thrown out the window. The relaxing music had been usurped by *Dr. Phil* on TV and I was in the spa bath with wet hair plastered across my face screaming like a banshee. Why was *Dr. Phil* even on? He wasn't part of the plan, or hypnobirthing, but I could barely find the strength to tell Mat to turn him off.

Up until this point I had been in labour for eight hours with no drugs. When the 'ring in' Obstetrician came in to check how dilated I was he announced it was just 3cm. You can imagine how far my heart sank then. 'WHAT THE FUCKING HYPNOBIRTH ARE YOU TALKING ABOUT?' I screamed – inside my head. Eight hours for 3cm? Is this a joke? I was devastated, and then – like delivering the knockout punch in a boxing match – he turned to the nurse in front of me and said, 'She'll need an epidural,' and walked out.

No No NO! This was not the plan. What is going on people? This is not how it was meant to be. I'm in so much pain, I'm devastated because I am not as strong as I thought I was, and I am being forced into taking a pain-relief road I didn't want to take. I hate needles and I'm about to have one inserted into my spine. I sob defeatedly into Mat's shoulder.

An hour later I am in spinal block heaven, asking myself why anyone would want to give birth naturally, when they could have the golden ticket of an epidural. (I wonder if I could get my hypnobirth fee back? Doubtful.) There are of course some negatives to having an epidural, and one of them is that you can't feel the contractions, so everything slows down. I had laboured another eight hours since I was given the epidural and throughout the day any time I began to feel more pain, my index finger would instinctively push the call button for a top up.

Thank God the midwife, who had my birth plan, had finished her shift. Sitting in bed watching TV and haphazardly hitting the call button for more drugs was quite contradictory to the original no drugs, peace, love and positive mantra-humming plan. I'm sure the staff saw countless first-time mums with rosy visions and careful preparations for their perfect birth. At least she didn't eye roll at me when I presented her with one of the three copies that I handed out to the team for this big holistic group effort. As a result of the magical epidural, I ended up pushing for another three and a half hours before eventually, at 10.36pm on 4 July, Oliver Jason Geoffrey Brumfitt was born. Mat's reaction to watching Oliver being delivered was priceless. He was crying and screaming, 'Oh my God, oh my God!' over and over. Later the obstetrician said he had never seen such an overwhelmed and animated reaction from a new father. I had only seen Mat cry on a few occasions. For the most part he likes to hold his cards close to his chest, but this moment was like every beautiful and joyous emotion that he had ever felt in his entire life was spilling out of his body. Seeing Mat so vulnerable and joyous made the moment even more special for me.

In my arms was my darling Oliver – tiny fingernails, wet jet black hair and perfect in every way. What a surreal moment. I was a mother. When I rang my parents to tell them the news, they raced into the hospital to meet their gorgeous grandson, and when they held him I remember thinking I hadn't seen them look that happy for such a long time. With tears in my eyes I introduced them to Oliver, and I nearly burst with pride and excitement when I announced his middle name – Jason.

Jason was my brother; he had passed away suddenly just five years earlier. I knew that new life in our family would help ease the pain of a lifelong sentence of grieving. The instant I held Oliver I knew I would die for him. It was only now that I understood the irreversible sadness within my mum. No matter what happens, or what is said, or what other joy she experiences in her life, it will never be pure. Her life will always be tainted, always, and so will my dad's. Only now holding Oliver in my arms do I understand the enormity of love and loss. It is a love I've never felt, it is beyond words.

It was close to midnight and I was shattered, Mum and Dad had left and I was stuffing my face with about twenty hospital sandwiches. (I have a strange penchant for hospital sandwiches, airplane bread rolls and seafood extender – tragic I know!) It was time to put my enormous breasts and equally gigantic nipples to the test. It was time to introduce Oliver to breastfeeding and boy did he like it. Instinctively he knew exactly what to do, unlike me, who was feeling quite bewildered by the entire situation. There was Mat standing to my right looking completely fascinated as if I was an animal doing something extraordinary on a David Attenborough special. There was the midwife, her hands squeezing my nipples encouraging the colostrum out and, of course, there was Oliver, savaging around my nipples like a stray dog in a garbage bin. Little Oliver, newest addition to the family and a new human being, made himself completely at home sucking on my nipples. Extraordinary. My nipples had never seen so much action. Within half an hour I was sore and he was sleepy and I thought to myself, I deserve a long hot shower.

My vagina was so sore from the birth that I could barely just waddle into the bathroom before easing myself down on to the commode chair. I turned on the tap and the feeling of hot water running down my back was magical. If it wasn't for the old person's chair I was sitting in, the institutional tiles, the handrails and the strip lighting, I'm sure the bathroom had the potential to feel like a day spa.

I then look down at my belly and I have my first (of many) WHAT THE FUCK? moments. What had been the most luscious, sexy and beautiful part of my body for the past nine months had degenerated into a blob. It was jelly-like, and wobbly and, quite frankly, revolting.

I remember when I first found out I was pregnant I was so delighted that at last my tummy, aka my 'trouble area,' was going to be justifiably big and round, and for the first time in my life I wouldn't have to suck it in. I had loved everything about my growing belly, the shape, the feel and, of course, the content! One of my favourite pastimes was rubbing soap all over my belly in the shower, around and around my hands would explore the new terrain; I had never felt more in love with my body than I did when I was pregnant.

So there I was, sitting in a commode chair, with nipples the size of dinner plates, a wobbly jelly belly, blood streaming from my vagina, exhausted, overwhelmed and about to take on the biggest challenge of my life. Things were never going to be the same again.

The next few days in hospital were a blur of sleeping, feeding and eating. I was so in love with Oliver, the love a mother has for her child is a love that you can't comprehend until you've experienced it; completely and utterly overwhelming. On Oliver's birth announcement cards I shared a poem by Maureen Hawkins that sums it up perfectly 'Before you were conceived I wanted you. Before you were born I loved you. Before you were here an hour, I would die for you. This is the miracle of life.'

Bringing Oliver home was magical, it was so lovely to see a baby in the big cot that had been sitting in an empty nursery for months. We settled into a really good routine and after a few weeks of staying indoors and lying low, it was time for Mat and I to make our debut back on to the social scene.

It was Saturday night.

Concealer under my dark eyes – check. Big grandma knickers holding everything together – check. Ollie fed, nursing bra stuffed with breast pads – check.

I finish straightening my hair and slipped my feet into a new pair of funky animal print flats. Animal print makes me happy and as I look at my reflection in the mirror I think to myself I look pretty good for a new mum with a 6-week-old baby.

We were going to our friends Viki and Mary for dinner, who conveniently live only two streets away from our home. We've been friends with these guys for what feels like a lifetime. I went to school with Mary's daughter, Kaija, so Mary and Viki have that extra nice feeling of being old family friends, and their place is a house you never want to leave, filled with laughter, good times and plenty of food. Their Latvian bread rolls, filled with bacon and onion are TO DIE FOR. Sometimes at Easter I will score a bag of them and hide them in the freezer, not tell the rest of the family and eat them all myself. How bad is that? You know what though, no one appreciates those bacon and onion rolls like I do, so I almost feel like it's my right to eat them all myself.

Visits to Mary and Viki's house always make me think of Salome, our Greek neighbour who lived across the road from our family home in Flagstaff Hill when I was growing up. I can remember sitting in Salome's kitchen, with its unique and appealing house smell, drinking Greek coffee and eating Turkish Delight. With an

Australian mother and a British father I've always enjoyed being friends with people from different cultures, partly because of the diversity of stories and ways of life, but mostly because of the food. We were a meat and three veg family and it always drove me up the wall. I wanted garlic, lemongrass, spices and herbs but the fanciest accompaniment I ever got to my plain food was tartar sauce on my fish. Don't get me wrong, I don't strategically go out of my way to make friends of different ethnicities just for the sake of my stomach, but I don't mind the added bonus of a good chicken korma with an Indian friend or a little bit of Asian pickle from my Chinese mates.

See how easily distracted I get from a story? Food will do it every time. Back to my straight hair and animal print shoes.

That evening we had a really good time at Mary and Viki's. It felt great to be out socialising and enjoy the sense of pride in having everyone oooing and ahhhing over our little creation, Oliver. With so many hands on deck I was even able to eat without interruption. The evening came to an end at about 9.30pm and Mat, Oliver and I commenced our very short walk home.

We'd been walking for no more than a minute when I got the urge to do a Number Two. Now before children I was one of these people that could go great distances at holding in a Number Two, and a Number One for that matter also. But on this evening, the urgency to do a Number Two came out of nowhere and was a force to be reckoned with. I turned to Mat and said,'I need to go to the toilet.' He pointed out we'd be home in a minute, clearly not sensing the urgency in my voice or the intensity in my eyes. 'Hun, I really need to do a Number Two, like NOW.' Finally Mat got it and began to walk faster. 'Oh fuck,' I gasped, 'Seriously I am going to shit my pants Mat. Run ahead, open up the house and turn off the alarm so I can run straight in!' And off he went, running ahead, me lagging behind, half running, half shuffling, definitely wincing, pushing the Bugaboo pram down the street. I always wonder what the neighbours must have thought if they'd seen us running with our new baby in the pram. Did they think, 'Oh look at that new family being healthy and active on a Saturday night'? No one would have thought, 'Oh look at that woman holding in a crap while her poor husband frantically runs ahead to make the house entry smooth and without delay.'

I made it to our street, running as fast as I could while remembering my new baby was in a pram that wasn't designed to be pushed at speed and on footpaths that were death traps for a newborn baby with developing fontanelles (you know, the soft bits of the head). I can see my home, my perfect white picket fence, that's where I live Number Two, here we go... I make it through the gate, through the front door and – just metres from the toilet – the relief of (almost) making it becomes too much and right there in the middle of the hallway, I shit my pants. In front of my husband. I shuffle my way to the toilet and fix myself up. I will spare you the details but let's just say that pooing your own pants as an adult is not only messy and gross, it is crushing for your self esteem.

When I reappeared Mat looked at me under his eyebrow and then, I can only assume out of embarrassment for me, turned away. I was completely and utterly mortified. Mat and I had always had a very open relationship, I could say and do most things in front of him and I know that his feelings wouldn't change. But pooing my pants in front of him was definitely new territory for our marriage.

Since the birth of Oliver, any feeling of being an object of desire, or having my own sexual inclinations had already been somewhat on the back burner. Standing there in my completely mortified state, wife to my gorgeous husband, left me feeling extremely undesirable. The thought of being his lover again was almost inconceivable. It was as if giving birth had flicked a switch off inside my head, and with poo in my pants and the look on his face, that switch wasn't getting turned back any time soon.

A few weeks after the Number Two incident I decided that I was going to be proactive about my body and fitness and it was time to get back onto the netball court. It seemed like the perfect sport to jump back into, I knew how to play and there was a crèche at the gym for child-minding emergencies.

As he was my first child, Oliver didn't see the inside of a crèche until Cruz, my second baby, came along two years later. Most first-time mums are pedantic about sleep schedules, avoiding germs and feeding regimes, and I was no different. It's funny how relaxed you are the more children you have. I remember a girlfriend of mine, Mel, laughing one day after we'd both had our second babies, a teething rusk fell on the pavement and I picked it up, said, 'ten second rule,' which basically means if it hasn't been on the ground for longer than ten seconds it's germ-free, and handed it back to the baby. We were reminiscing about the days when we'd just had our first babies, when that would have been a cardinal sin!

Anyway, I digress. So on this Tuesday morning I was delighted to have some time to myself, out on the netball court, getting some exercise and playing a sport I've played and loved for over twenty years. Without sounding too cocky, I'd like to think I'm a good netballer. Being highly competitive from a young age, it was always my ambition to be the best, and I nearly was until I discovered smoking and the odd illegal underage drink with friends. I was about sixteen when I took a break from netball, I played for the best club in the state, and if I had stuck at it, I am sure I would've gone all the way. But from a 16-year-old's perspective, a white cider in the park with my mates seemed like such a great alternative to netball practice.

So, you might say that showing off my talents at a casual recreational game of netball at 10.10am on a Tuesday morning was going to be like a come back of sorts. After the first quarter I felt on top of the world, I'd taken a couple of intercepts and I was able to sprint up and down the court playing the centre position with speed and agility. I still had it, and I was pumped as I headed back on to the court for the second quarter.

As centre, I start with the ball and pass ideally to the wing attack. She then usually passes to the goal shooter who hopefully will score. As planned, this took place but the shooter missed the goal and therefore the opposing team had the ball. I raced down to catch my centre opponent and the ball was making its way down the court. Like a movie inside my head, I knew what was going to happen and saw my opportunity to take a speccy (SPECTACULAR) intercept. Sure enough, the girl that took the ball passed to the girl I knew she would pass to and BOOM, super-speedy me took a dazzling intercept and I had the ball. Bravo me.

Hang on, what is that warm liquid running down my leg? Oh fuck me, I've just wet myself. Mortified. I quickly pass the ball, do this kind of scraping motion with my shoe to the slight bit of wee that has hit the court, and use the dry leg to sort of awkwardly wipe the wet leg so it's not glistening for all to see. Inside my head I am thinking to myself, 'What, no wait, let me rephrase that... WHAT just happened?'

The entire way through my pregnancy my very good girlfriend Nikki, who is a physiotherapist, would quiz me on whether I'd been doing my pelvic floor exercises, to which I would always dismissively lie, 'Yep, I am doing them right now.'

Why, why, why had I not used all that spare time I had before children to take five minutes out of my day to do the exercises? It's okay, I have the answer, because until you have children you think you have no time, it's only after you have them you realise that you were living the 'abundance of time on your hands' dream.

I managed to get through to the end of the match but it's fair to say that there was nothing speccy about my game in those last couple of quarters. The girls on the court must have assumed I'd run out of steam and gone too hard too soon. I'm sure they thought, 'Where's Mrs Cocky Pants now, sprinting around with her bouncy pony tail and dazzling intercepts?'

We lost the game, I lost my dignity and with my tail between my legs I drove back to my mum's house, where she was looking after Ollie. I took my near exploding boobs out of my hideous and painful sports bra and sat there on the couch, milk dripping from my nipples as Oliver latched on, and I explained to Mum what happened. She suggested I wear sanitary pads for my next game, which I did. In fact I wore two pads and three pairs of knickers for the next month of matches. One pad on knickers, followed by another ensemble of pad and knickers, finished off with the ultimate 'keep it all in and let nothing out' Nancy Ganz-style, bad boy knickers.

I was determined to never let another drop of urine hit the netball court, and it didn't. But of course it was never going to, because I never allowed myself to play as hard as I'd always done. I didn't trust my body anymore.

CHAPTER THREE

Growing up

WHEN I WAS GROWING UP I never hated my body or felt like I couldn't trust it. I went through the usual ups and downs of being a teenager, I tried diets, I sometimes ate rice cakes and tuna for a week, I had days when I was convinced I was fat, I experimented with stuff, but was basically okay.

Reflecting on my childhood, I think I was too caught up in surviving bullying to worry about my body. I was bullied during primary and high school. My first memory of being bullied was in Year 5, when I suddenly got a lot of attention from the boys and quite simply the girls didn't like it. I remember being called a slut and not understanding why, I never sought out the boys' attention, it just happened to come my way.

Heading into high school was daunting but I soon found my groove and had a very close circle of friends. For the first time in a long time I felt protected. One of my best friends was Katarina Urban, she was so freaking cool. When we weren't pulling up our white socks only to scrunch them straight back down with our super-short summer school uniforms, we were smoking behind the deli, watching Stephen King movies or experimenting with weird séances. I felt like I had finally found someone who 'got me', and then my parents declared we were moving and I would need to go to a new school. I was as equally devastated as I was excited, a fresh start was going to be fun, I could reinvent who I was and become the 'cool new girl'. I had it all planned.

So when I started at Unley High, with my perfect uniform, perfect hair and shiny shoes, I had no idea what I was walking into. Starting half way through Year 10, groups and alliances had been formed and I felt extremely awkward. The spotlight was on me, people wanted to know who I was, where I came from and what group I would fit into. Like most schools there was the cool club of kids, the Italians, the geeks and the Greeks while the in-betweeners (not cool but not geeks), mostly just flew under the radar. Of course I wanted to be in the cool kids club, the ones whose uniforms pushed the boundaries of acceptable, who smoked at recess and lunch, and who didn't give me too much attention in those first few weeks. When casual day was announced, I thought I'd found my opportunity to set the record straight, I am going to smash my coolness out the park and finally the cool group would claim me as their own.

Mum took me shopping to Sportsgirl – a clothing shop for young girls – whose signature t-shirt with multi-coloured writing, tucked into a pair of 501 jeans, was going to catapult me into the realms of the cool club. Sportsgirl had advertisements on TV that ended with a woman's voice whispering 'Sportsgirl' that sounded like a person breathing out and saying 'Spooooortsgiiiiiirl' at the same time. I thought it was brilliant.

The night before casual day I laid my clothes out on the floor, so excited that I was going to be able to express who I was and ooze coolness from every one of my pores. When I arrived at school it became apparent that I was not in Kansas anymore – I had completely missed the brief, everyone else was wearing LaCoste jumpers, mostly all the same type but in different colours, or Mambo jumpers. I didn't fit in. Up until this day if my fate at the school was undetermined it became very apparent by recess that I was to be outcast, I was not 'in', in fact I was very much alone.

The mean girl that led the charge in my demise was named Edith (Eddy for short). She was a solid girl, one that you wouldn't want to get into a physical stoush with, and she was mean. Mean, nasty, cruel. Basically she made my life hell with her posse of other mean girls, and on occasions I was really frightened she was going to physically hurt me.

She would threaten me and I would often overhear rumours going around the school that she wanted to 'bash me'. She frightened the life out of me, I guess it comes as no surprise that I chose to do boxing at the gym as my work experience – looking back now with my wise adult perception I was probably just thinking of finding a way to protect myself if she did ever come after me.

It's only been in recent years, since having children, that I have softened the ambition I've nursed that if I saw her I'd like to punch her in the head and flatten her with a roundhouse. For a long time, if she ever came up in conversation or if I saw her name on Facebook, I couldn't help but feel I wanted some sort of revenge. But of course now that I am an adult I have a better understanding of why bullies bully, I am sure she suffered herself, and maybe picking on me made herself feel better about her own situation.

Kids can be cruel, and often the guys would sing a song about Eddy along the lines of, 'Edith Eddy likes to give heady.' The boys would often torment Eddy about the fact she liked giving 'headjobs', otherwise known as blow jobs, she would laugh it off, but there were also times she acted like she was proud of the headjob reputation. The poor girl probably gave a guy a blowjob once and he took it upon himself to tell all his mates, next thing, she is universally labelled as a slut.

It kind of reminds me of all the times I rejected men throughout my life, only to be called a slut within a second of the rejection. Conversations would often go like this,

'Hey beautiful, can I buy you a drink?'

'No thanks, I'm just waiting for a friend.'

'Fucking slut,' under the breath.

What the? I know many women will relate to this. I remember another occasion at my old high school some older kid tried to kiss me, and when I rejected him, he called me a slut. He got his just desserts when Jason found out, Jason and his mates in their car tried to run him off his bike. A little over the top and protective – yes, but suffice it to say he never called me a slut again.

Anyway, back to Eddy. She was a nasty pasty but I am sure she had her own story too. Something or someone influenced her to be like this, I don't blame her (now) and I don't feel resentment like I used to. It is what it is – just another story that shaped the person I am now. At the time though, it was more difficult to be philosophical about the daily taunts and mean-spirited comments. The way I was treated then still impacts on me to this day. A few years ago a couple of my girlfriends went to the movies together and didn't invite me. Mat was away travelling at the time and I was deeply hurt that they didn't stop to think that it might have been nice for me to go too. Instead of just brushing it out as 'no big deal.' I created a huge deal about it, sending my friends a ranty email about how 'excluded' I felt and questioning our friendship. Only on reflection of the embarrassing way I behaved was I able to see the truth, depth and meaning of my actions. It wasn't about the movies, it was about being transported back to that place of feeling 'unwanted' and 'left out', just like in high school. Thank goodness I've been able to come to terms with those feelings now, after all there is nothing worse than a 'needy' friend.

Getting bullied was tough, I still think about it to this day, but there was something else that made a much bigger impact on my childhood and on the person that I am today – death.

Death has shaped me in good ways and in bad, but mostly good, I think. I have always been an impatient person, I loathe the saying 'Rome wasn't built in a day', for me everything has to be done yesterday. I'm sure it's one of my most annoying traits for close family and friends, because wheels always have to be in motion, we must be moving forward, there is no time to chill out and relax, because, as I explain to them, life is short. Which actually translates to, 'Death is imminent, we could be taken at any time.'

Growing up I had firsthand experience with death and tragedy. I was fifteen, it was Christmas Eve, 1994, when we received a strange phone call at home. Dad answered and a man said, 'Do you know Keith Butterworth?' Dad said he did, and then the call was disconnected. Uncle Keith, a gently spoken, calm and kind man, was my dad's brother. Dad was puzzled by the phone call, but a few minutes later there was a knock at the front door. It was two detectives.

They explained that Uncle Keith and Catherine – his long term girlfriend – had both gone missing. It was completely bizarre and didn't make sense. Information was limited and when they left all we really knew was that both Keith and Catherine were missing, and that the circumstances of their disappearance were slightly odd.

The next day was Christmas Day and Mum, Dad and I were going to Fiji for a holiday. Jason was nearly twenty and Justine, my older sister, was twenty-three, and both had other commitments. Even though I was a slightly snitchy teenager, I was looking forward to spending some time with Mum and Dad, getting spoilt like an only child.

We arrived in Fiji and Mum and Dad were ringing back home every few hours to find out if there was any news. They protected me from most of the discussions but I certainly sensed that something was not right and bad news was coming. I was walking on the beach with Mum on 27 December when she told me to expect the worst. A day later on my sixteenth birthday we found out that Uncle Keith was dead, and that he had killed Catherine. The significance of the words, 'You must expect the worst,' followed up with the worst actually happening, has been one of my biggest hurdles to overcome. It was almost like those words were anchored into my psyche and all future decisions that I made were based on the notion that the worst could and would happen.

While in Fiji we had come across a couple on their honeymoon, Kelley and Eric. You know in those big resorts how you keep seeing the same people and eventually you feel you can say hello, and start up a conversation. This particular couple were very special. During the time that we'd been in Fiji Mum or Dad must have told them about the situation back home, so when the terrible news came, Kelley and Eric offered support and insisted on helping us get back home as soon as we could. Mum and Dad had trouble getting flights out of Fiji, so Kelley and Eric, who had contacts in the airline industry, spent hours on the phone helping us to secure flights. Doing all this, on their honeymoon. I remember having a walk with Eric on the beach, we chatted and it felt like I'd known him a lifetime, he even gave me a cigarette to smoke, which made him feel incredibly uncomfortable because he knew my folks would be less than impressed.

On the ground back home, my Grandma (Dad's mum) had lost her son and was trying to support my sister and brother at our family home. Apparently there were many reporters coming to the house and harassing them for comments on the circumstances of Uncle Keith and Catherine's death. On the front cover of the *Sunday Mail* (Adelaide's major paper) was a full-page picture of Uncle Keith's face.

It was horrible, and so were the circumstances of their death. Uncle Keith had strangled Catherine and then driven himself out to an empty paddock north of the city and killed himself by inhaling the carbon monoxide from his car. Life as I knew it, from the age of sixteen, became unpredictable and the notion that bad things were going to happen became a way of life for me. Jason's death several years later validated this. Whenever I was with a guy, he was going to cheat and leave me. Something bad was always going to happen to those I loved.

There was some goodness that came from the terrible situation though and that was my lifelong friendship with Kelley. After arriving home in Adelaide I wanted to keep in contact with Kelley and Eric, and I often sent them a letter in the mail or rang them for a chat on the phone. We certainly hadn't established a friendship that would justify me rocking up on their doorstep with a bag and in need of a place to stay about a year after we'd first met, but that's exactly what I did. One evening I had a fight with Mum and Dad (I don't even recall what it was about) and I packed a bag and left. I went and stayed at a girlfriend's house and then the next day with just a few items in a bag and a few packets of ciggies, I jumped on the 7am bus to Melbourne. When I rang my mum the next day she was beside herself and shouted, 'WHERE ARE YOU?' to which I replied, 'Melbourne.' Poor Mum and poor Dad. I was a temperamental teenager and they were and still are the most kind and thoughtful parents anyone could ever wish for.

So I needed a place to stay, I had no plans, the world was my oyster and I was in the big smoke! Kelley and Eric had a six-month-old baby by this stage, Rickel, and there I was – a thoughtless, reckless, and most definitely selfish teen – thinking it would be appropriate to come and stay. And stay I did, not for a week, or even a fortnight but for six months. Yes you read that correctly, six months – to all the mums out there, could you imagine a teenager, with not much sense of anything except their own needs, crashing in your place when you've just started a family?

Kelley and I still joke about my selfishness to this day. How our lives have changed so much. Our friendship is my most treasured, she has been a sister, a mother and a best friend to me. She has been there for me during all the good times and the bad, and I've had the great pleasure of watching her three children grow up. I sometimes wonder if I'll ever get one of her children wanting to come stay with me – I think she's probably advised them against it though, who would want to come stay in a house with my three noisy kids!

I stayed in Melbourne for about a year and worked in cafés and restaurants. Because I had dropped out of school (partly because of the bullying) I was not qualified to do anything. Washing dishes seemed quite attractive when I was sixteen but what was I going to do for the rest of my life? I was glad in the end to move back to Adelaide, to be 'at home' again, but the future looked pretty bleak.

I spent the next few years working in every job imaginable. I worked in a nursing home (still my favourite job to this day, I adored looking after people), at juice bars and coffee shops, I worked as a nanny, I pretended to be a receptionist for about two days and I worked as security in nightclubs. I also spent some time travelling. On my 21st birthday I set off on a backpacking adventure through Europe but actually only made it to London, where I got a job that paid enough to go visiting random places like Tunisia and Corfu (because of the cheap discounts), and never used my backpack once!

When I came back to Australia I finally found my feet. I applied for a job in sales at a hotel marketing company and gradually climbed my way up. (Cue music 'She works hard for her money'.) I eventually found myself in the position of Operations Manager for Australia and New Zealand and was living in the beautiful city of Christchurch.

I had a small apartment on the second floor of a six-floor apartment block just a ten minute walk from the city centre and my office. Hagley Park was a few footsteps away and there was a Chinese restaurant down the end of my street, I even had a karaoke system set up in my teeny tiny apartment, which in hindsight makes me cringe, the poor neighbours had to listen to me belting out endless Madonna and Wham tunes. (There is no holding back a girl who had her childhood in the 1980s).

I was in my mid twenties, I had a great job, no financial commitments, (I didn't even have a car), and I felt like I had my entire life ahead of me. I was in my prime and I bloody knew it, which really is the key to extracting all of the enjoyment out of life. A good life is too often wasted on people who don't appreciate what they've got, so I felt particularly chuffed to be living the dream but being awake at the same time. My weekdays revolved around work, which I loved, and the weekends were dedicated to karaoke, shopping, Eggs Benedict. I didn't have a lot of friends in Christchurch; in fact it's probably fair to say I had just one – Janet.

I had found it hard to make new friends in Christchurch. I worked with a diverse bunch of about thirty people, but because I was 'the boss' I didn't extend the friendship branch because I didn't want to blur the lines. I had already done that with one male employee and let's just say it didn't end well. But Janet was different, she had been working in the call centre for about seven years and she was older and wiser than most (around forty) and from the second I arrived she took me under her wing and gave me the support and guidance I so often didn't think I needed. (But of course I did).

Janet had short blonde hair, drove a bright yellow MR2, smoked far too many cigarettes and drank as much coffee as I did. Every time she'd say six (sux) or dick (duck) I would laugh so hard. That came out wrong, we didn't often have conversations about six dicks, but I'm sure you catch my drift. Without dedicating an entire chapter to Janet you'll have to take my word for it when I say that Janet Scott was a bloody good egg and we like her a lot.

The morning of 2 May started like any other. The alarm went off, I dragged myself to the shower, applied my makeup and styled my hair. I had recently cut all my hair off and the styling stole an annoying amount of my precious time in the morning. A few weeks earlier I had walked into a hair salon with luscious long blonde locks and announced that I wanted to chop it all off, just like Victoria Beckham on her wedding day. You should have seen the hairdresser's face, it was like she'd just struck gold, and I think it might have been the highlight of her career to date. She cut off almost fifteen inches and enjoyed every minute of it. I'm not sure if I looked better with a brown pixie hairdo, but one thing I know for sure the faffing around to get the fringe bit right in the mornings was beyond irritating. So, hair and makeup done, perfectly coordinated dress and heels on, I headed downstairs to get picked up by Janet. With both of us sucking back on ciggies, music pumping in the yellow beast, off to work we went. I'm sure we looked quite tragic but in those short car rides to the office, we owned whatever we thought we owned at the time. It was always easy and laid back with Janet, we were always just us doing our thing with the occasional little bit of Janet's friendly (sort of) road rage thrown into the mix.

It was about an hour after we'd arrived at work when the phone rang, Janet took the call and asked me for some privacy, which was slightly odd because it was my office that she was in. I went and sat in the sales room and watched her take the call through the glass that separated the two offices. I wondered who she was talking to; it was obvious that it was something quite serious because the look on her face is one I will never forget. After a few minutes she beckoned me back into the office. 'You need to take this call,' she said to me. I took the phone and pressed it to my ear. It was my sister.

Oh dear God, oh fuck what is wrong with Mum and Dad. Has Dad had a heart attack? Oh God, what is it? 'Taryn, I have some bad news,' said my sister. 'Jason is dead.' I drop the phone, I scream uncontrollably. 'NO NO NONONONONONO.' I can no longer hold up the weight of my body. I collapse to the floor sobbing uncontrollably. I still can't recall what happened next, I know there was a conversation about flights home but it all became a blur.

The next thing I properly remember is smoking a cigarette outside and drinking a coffee with Janet. I felt so numb. I watched people as they walked past me. Life was continuing to happen as normal and it made me want to scream. I remember feeling so confused and so angry. Why is the world still moving? Why are people still doing? Don't you fucking people know that Jason Butterworth is DEAD?

I'd decided I would be okay to fly home to Adelaide alone, but Justine my sister insisted I go to the doctors and get some valium to help keep me calm during the journey. Janet took me to the doctor then back to my apartment to grab some personal items and then she drove me to the airport.

Boarding that flight alone was harder than I thought. I remember I had a spare seat next to me and on the other side was a middle-aged business man. He looked less than friendly when what I needed was someone to give me a hug, or at least a kindly look. He was definitely not the guy to give me what I needed. I felt like I was drowning and no one around me knew the insurmountable grief I was feeling, I found it hard to fill my lungs with oxygen, my chest was tight, I felt nauseous. Watching the clouds float past the window of the aeroplane was eerie. Where is Jason right now? Who is he with? What is he doing? And true to form I start thinking about where his body was. Is he naked and cold lying on a metal bed in one of those drawer things you pull out at the morgue? How white is he? Are his lips blue? Is his body stiff? This is too weird; none of what I am thinking is making sense. Is it the valium or are these thoughts normal? I didn't know.

After a change in Melbourne I arrived in Adelaide and was picked up by my sister. At home the house was full of well-meaning friends and neighbours wanting to help, but I just wanted to be alone with my family. My mum was still sedated; both she and my father were incoherent with shock and grief.

My parents adored Jason; he was their only son and quite a character. He was charming, funny, charismatic, and a heroin addict, and at twenty-seven years of age on a park bench in Sydney's Belmore Park he had injected heroin into his veins and took his last breath. He was all alone.

CHAPTER FOUR

Frilled neck lizards

AS WE DROVE UP GOODWOOD ROAD in a black limousine heading to Jason's funeral I remember looking at my mum's face and thinking how beautiful she looked. In fact I can't recall another occasion that she looked as pretty as she looked that day.

It had been years since I'd considered my mum to be 'pretty'. Not because she's not of course, but it's not a regular thought that a young woman in her twenties has about her mother. I remember as a child watching her get ready to go out with my dad and thinking how beautiful she was. I can remember the smell of her perfume and her hair as she kissed me goodbye. She was so pretty, I loved her clothes, I loved her shoes and I loved her sparkling jewellery.

Sitting in the limousine opposite me was a mother whose soul had been ripped out. She was enduring the worst pain and suffering of all – that of losing a child. So why did she look so pretty? I've never asked her but I wonder if she felt that she needed to look pretty for Jason?

We always knew that Jason was well loved among his peers but I think there was part of us that felt concerned about how many people would be at his funeral. It was an unspoken concern but I just knew there was an element of uncertainty. Jason had been living like a nomad in the years leading up to his death, and hadn't spent much time in Adelaide, so it was likely that a lot of people he had known wouldn't be there. How wrong we were. There were over two hundred people at the service – old faces, kindly friends, tennis friends, family friends and of course his school friends. It was the most beautiful and comforting thing to see so many people there remembering Jason and giving us support.

My sister Justine and I had written a few words about Jason to share at the funeral. I didn't know how I was going to get through the eulogy without breaking down, but I dare say that the content of my piece might've helped me to keep on track. I just had to tell this story.

Justine, Jason and I grew up in Flagstaff Hill, about 20km out of the city, in a new estate of houses. There was lots of space, and we had a great park right across from our street. Our weekends were filled with bike rides, playing on zip lines, and trying to avoid getting swooped by magpies. The magpies were really aggressive, especially when we were on our bikes (no helmets, it was the '80s after all) cycling up and down the big dipper at the park. One day Jason came home with blood dripping down from his yellow blonde hair. We all thought he'd fallen off his bike, but he'd been badly pecked by a magpie. I tried to explain to Cruz just a few years ago that his Uncle Jason (who of course he had never met) had died because he 'had something' that made him sick, Cruz exclaimed with absolute certainty in his voice, 'No he didn't, Jason got pecked by the magpies and died.' Somehow in his five years of life he must've overheard the magpie story and correlated it to Jason's death.

There were not only a lot of magpies at Flagstaff Hill, there were also a lot of snakes, skinks and lizards, and every weekend without fail Jason and I would jump over the back fence and head into the gorge to go seek out the wildlife. We spent many hours adventuring together, lifting bark off trees looking for geckos, and trying not to get cut up by the barbed wire as we adventured into places we probably shouldn't have been. We went yabbying (catching crayfish), we caught tadpoles, frogs, loads of lizards and once, to our mum's absolute horror, we caught a baby brown snake. But the best reptile we ever came across was a frilled neck lizard.

Catching a frilled neck lizard was the story that I told at Jason's funeral. I could have told the story about how he ran beside me encouraging me to the finish of an 800m run at the State championships when I was ready to give up, I could have told the congregation how proud I was that Jason played Sean Penn's movie double in *The Thin Red Line*, I could have told many stories, but I just knew the frilled neck lizard story was the one that would have made him laugh.

My stomach was doing flips as I walked up to the podium to speak, I had to walk past the coffin and I felt overwhelmed as I visualised Jason lying in there. A few days earlier I had been to Jason's viewing with my family. It is to this day the hardest and most emotional thing I have ever done. I remember the frosting on the door of the funeral parlour and how the blurred coffin came in to focus very quickly as the funeral director opened the door. I remember being last to walk over to the coffin, I had never felt more petrified in all my life. My heart was ripped out of my chest that day as I watched my parents go to Jason, talking to him like he was alive, sobbing and calling his name... I remember my dad's strong old hands caressing Jason's cheeks just as he would've done twenty-seven years earlier when he was a little baby. I remember my mum touching Jason's hair. For some strange reason I was almost convinced that he would jump out of the coffin and say BOO! That sounds weird but when you've had an older sibling that you've spent the best part of your life fighting with, playing jokes on and teasing, it would seem almost possible – except it wasn't going to. He was very, very dead. His skin was cold and white and his body was stiff and hard. I touched his chest and I felt something underneath his clothes, like crepe paper, I later found out it was bandaging from the autopsy.

My brother – dead, cold, hard, and lying in coffin.

So as I walked past the coffin on the day of the funeral there was no illusion in my head that what was inside was anything other than horrifying. I'd seen the body, it scared me, it didn't comfort me, there wasn't closure, I simply saw my brother dead, and it's a memory that will never leave my mind.

I had to stay focused on telling a really good story, for Jason and the people who loved him. So I explained to the crowd of friends and family how we'd been out on one of our regular adventures and on this particular day, when I was six and Jason was ten, we had come across a frilled neck lizard. I think what Jason and I liked best about this particular reptile was that when we confronted it, rather than trying to scamper away like most of the skinks and lizards, the frilled neck held its ground and with fierce eyes and a hissing tongue, it was ready to defend its position.

These particular lizards aren't exactly small, the average length of a frilled neck is 85cm, so effectively if you flipped the lizard's body length from horizontal to vertical, it would have towered over me. It gets its name from the large ruff of skin that usually lies folded back against its head and neck. When the lizard is frightened, it opens its mouth really wide, spreads out its frill, displaying bright red and orange scales, and raises its body, sometimes holding its tail above its body. We had come face to face with the king of the gorge.

Most people coming across this lizard would probably run the other way, but not us, and I wasn't scared either, because I was with my big brother.

Some days we could walk for hours in one direction and would be a long way from home. Luckily this day we were near enough that I (the rookie/apprentice) could run back as instructed and grab the red tub. I crept slowly back from the lizard and then as soon as it was safe, bolted as fast as I could back home, through the barbed wire, and over the back fence. The sense of urgency and excitement was almost too much to bear. Those were the best years of my life, so many highs and all for the right reasons.

I hurtled back with my red tub and we somehow managed to round that feisty and ferocious lizard into our big red tub. Holding the tub between us, Jason and I made it home, walking right around the block to the front of our house, because we couldn't get the tub over the back fence, sneaking it through the house and into the backyard.

Once we had got it there we got it some water, and then we decided the poor lizard must be hungry. We searched the fridge for food and came to the (very logical we thought at the time) conclusion that he/she would like red jelly. But how would we get the wobbly jelly into the lizards mouth? Jason came up with a great solution. We would use a thin white plumber's pipe, load it with jelly, point it at the lizard, and with a 'pufft' of air from our mouths, we would shoot the jelly directly down its throat. With its mouth open, its frill flared and red jelly sitting on its tongue in his mouth, we decided the mission was complete.

As I told this story at Jason's funeral I looked around the room at the many familiar faces and I knew there would be many stories out there about things that Jason had done and the adventures he got up to. Seeing some of Jason's friends that I hadn't seen for years gave me painful reminders of some of the best moments in my life. Like a fast rolling movie in my head, I could see Jason's life unfolding in my mind. We had the best childhood; holidays to America, Disneyland, New Zealand, and the Blue Mountains. Running through the sprinklers eating ice-blocks. Zinc cream on our noses at the beach. Justine, Jason and I playing 'runbacks' (when you were supposed to be in bed but would run down as close as you could to where Mum and Dad were watching TV without getting caught). School formals, first driving lessons, catching fish, we did it all. Our family life was good, and now it had ended. No more Jason. He was dead, he was gone, I no longer had a brother.

After the funeral we were given cups of coffee and plain biscuits. A funeral is always going to bring out the emotional eater in anyone. Someone should write a letter to the funeral homes and let them know if they want more business, stop running poxy advertisements on TV and start feeding mourners chocolate, and cream buns, maybe even pizza. Please just give us more than plain biscuits because I can tell you right now, we need it.

After some stilted conversations and a biscuit or three, it was time to head back to my parents' house to eat sandwiches cut into triangles and drink more coffee. It was here that a familiar face caught my eye. Mathew Brumfitt. Mat, Matty, or 'Crumpet' as his friends called him, had always managed to catch my eye. Mat and I had known each other for our entire lives. Our parents lived next door to each other before I was born, I've even got photos of Mat and Jason as babies lying on a rug next to each other. When Jason and his mates were teenagers, four years older than me, I was the annoying little sister. When the boys came over to our house to hang out, listen to music or swim I just couldn't help but attempt to infiltrate their world. I thought they were so cool. Mat, was always the stand out for me, he was shorter than the rest of them, stocky, with long hair and slight acne scars on his face that made him look like a bad boy. He was just my cup of tea. But I was Taryn Butterworth, Jason's younger sister, and all bets were off.

So at the wake when Mathew Brumfitt walked into Jason's room where I was standing flicking through books from the bookshelf, I was taken aback. It had been years since I'd seen him but he really hadn't changed much, in fact, I thought, he had improved. He had more style, and he was looking at me differently. I was a woman and he was a man and there was some kind of feeling between us, call if chemistry if you will.

I cut straight to the chase, asking Mat the kind of questions you would ask if you were sussing out a potential partner, 'What do you do for a crust?' 'Soooooo do you want children?' 'Do you like animals?' The answers were perfect, he was a custom's broker for an international shipping company, he did want children, and yes he liked animals. Winner, winner, chicken dinner, I was in, I had found my future husband.

We danced through another ten minutes of politely disguised interrogation of one another before I pulled the pin. After all it was Jason's wake and picking up one of his best mates didn't feel like the right thing to do.

The day after the wake I had a burning desire to contact Mat. I was only in Adelaide for another week before I needed to head back to my life in Christchurch. I decided I would go old school – write a letter and drop it off in his letterbox. This is what I wrote:

Dear Mathew

This letter is completely out of left field, and I apologise in advance for probably freaking you out. After seeing you yesterday, it brought back some feelings that I've had for a long time. I will be entirely honest and admit that I've had a 'crush' (hate that word!) on you for all my life.

I hope that you are sitting down right now because that comment has probably come as a bit of a shock to you. There is no doubt in my mind or anyone else's mind, that I am at a very fragile stage of my life, and what has happened to Jason probably has something to do with me writing this. It's not that I think anything will happen between us, I guess it just feels important to me that you know how I feel about you. It's crazy, I know, but my instincts tell me that I'm doing the right thing by letting you know – usually my instincts are right?

I know that you have a girlfriend, and I apologise for disrespecting her with this letter. I'm hoping you will keep it to yourself. I hope I haven't made you feel uncomfortable, if anything, perhaps you could feel flattered.

Thank you for being a great friend to Jason, he thought you were great.

If I don't see you before, I'm sure we'll see each other again in a few years, you'll be married and I'll have kids, and we'll both laugh about this letter!

Take care. Keep smiling

Love Taryn Butterworth

I remember exactly what I was hoping and thinking when I wrote that last sentence. That we would 'laugh' about it because we would be married to each other and we'd have kids together.

The next day I received a letter from Mat. It basically said that he was a little shocked to receive the letter but he was flattered and would like to see me before I headed back to New Zealand! As I read his letter my stomach was doing cartwheels. My immediate thought was when can I ring? Be cool Taryn, be cool, play it cool, remember what your mum always said, 'Make them want you more than you want them.' Good idea in theory, but impossible (for me) in reality.

As much as I tried to persuade myself with inner dialogue to wait, the urge was too strong and within just seconds of getting the letter my fingers were dialling his number.

Mat and I arranged to meet at The Unley on Clyde, a local pub just around the corner from Mum and Dad's place. We spoke for hours and hours and hours. I looked for cracks, I asked tough questions but he was exquisitely perfect. Could this really be happening? Our 'informal' date ended with a kiss and I just knew as I lay my head down on the pillow that night that this was the beginning of something very special.

It broke my heart a couple of days later when I had to leave my parents and head back to Christchurch on my own. I had to return to work, I had to pick up my life where I had left it a couple of weeks earlier. Janet insisted I stay with her for a week just to find my feet again and it was a welcome distraction. She took good care of me – home-cooked meals, electric blanket on the bed, all the good things in life – but eventually I had to go back to my empty apartment. The good vibes of Chinese take-away and fun times singing karaoke were replaced with silence and fear.

For the first time in my life, I hated being on my own. I was having nightmares nearly every night, and waking up crying and screaming with no one to console you isn't much fun. The silence in the apartment felt eerie. Jason was 'on the other side', I often wondered if he was looking down on me. Was he near me? Was he there? One night I put pen to paper and wrote a song. From the minute the pen touched the paper until the last word, it flowed, it was effortless and it most definitely felt like I had a helping hand.

Trying to find some inspiration from the tragedy that is,

Looking in all the wrong places all I can see is his.

His eyes, his smile

and the way we used to talk

His eyes, his smile

and how I gave him little thought.

Regret is something easily done
would those choices be the same?
If I could turn back the hands of time
would I do it different again?

His eyes, his smile
and the way we would play games
as a child, I watched him grow
things will never be the same.

I love him more each and every day
and I accept the life that he chose
He made his choices, he made his pain
but I forgive him... I suppose.

Jason, I love you
now your demons are all gone
since your death, I've felt such pain
but I know that you live on.

I know it's no Grammy award winner but it was never intended to be. In fact the night I wrote it I didn't have any expectations or intentions at all. I simply picked up a pen and it all came out.

The night I wrote the song was one of the very few occasions I felt at peace with Jason's death. Every other moment was a struggle and I felt quite broken and alone, I was scared at night on my own, I wasn't eating well and my heart belonged to someone else in another country. I wanted my mum and dad, I needed my family, Grieving on my own was too hard, I needed to come back to Adelaide. And so I did.

CHAPTER FIVE

My body image story

GETTING BULLIED WHEN I WAS GROWING UP didn't leave much time for worrying about my body, and I went through my teens and twenties with a relatively positive body image.

So once I'd had Oliver, shat my pants and wet myself, I was facing unknown territory about my relationship with my body. For the first time in my life, I felt that my body was betraying me. While there were many times throughout my life that I didn't like my body (when I was overweight) I was always able to accept responsibility and make the necessary changes to get back on track. But when I tried to get my body back into the shape it was in before I had Oliver, it wouldn't budge. I got frustrated. Really frustrated. For someone who likes control, being out of it wasn't much fun.

With a new healthy baby I should have been on top of the world, but there was something weighing me down, the thoughts I was having about my disgusting and hideous body. The jelly belly, angry looking, red stretch marks all over my tummy, and nipples the size of dinner plates. And to top it all off I was surrounded by images in magazines with headlines such as 'Baby bliss', 'How I got my body back' and 'Sexy new Mums'. What? Sex and new mothers in the same sentence, this can't be right?

Speaking of sex, I remember one of the first times after childbirth that I got 'back on the wagon' so to speak, it was a disaster. A disaster for me, not for Mat of course. Through many years of talking to friends about the subject of men and sex I have come to the conclusion that sex is, for men, just that. It doesn't matter if you don't have makeup on, just had an argument, or you haven't showered. Sex is good anytime, day or night. Women, on the other hand, are a little more complex, well I am anyway. So for sex to be on the radar for me, the time has to be right and I have to feel connected to Mat, otherwise it's like trying to fit a round peg in a square hole, it's just not going to work.

So back to my disastrous sex story. Everything was going smoothly until I hopped on top. Having sex on the side you can hide the belly, doggy style nothing can be seen, but on top, you are completely exposed. So there I was, not exactly riding Mat like I used to, but I was indeed back on the horse, I ensured my body was super straight, the taller I was the more stretched out my stomach was and the better it looked. I got carried away in the moment, I bent down to kiss Mat on the lips but before my lips met his, my stomach spilled out on top of his. In my head I was thinking how disgusting I must've looked. And of course as soon as those thoughts of 'what I looked like' popped into my head, the mojo was gone. Any ambition of an orgasm – gone. And to top it off, when I quickly sat back up and resumed my tall position, I noticed that my boobs were leaking milk.

There were many highs in those first few months of being a mum, I truly adored it and I was deliriously in love with Oliver. Motherhood was everything that I wanted it to be with a dose of extras that I didn't expect.

I spent the next fifteen months battling hard with the unrelenting ping pong conversation in my head, which kept informing me that I was fat, disgusting, gross and a complete sexual turn-off, and then just before my body image issues became a mental health issue, I was pregnant again, this time with Cruz.

Phew. I could now pretend that my hotdog stomach was an early sign of a growing baby and I was heading back into a world of pregnancy and a big delightful growing tummy. My jelly belly was going to be round and beautiful again. All feelings of being sad and sorry about the way I looked disappeared. I was now a vessel, my body had a purpose and all I needed to focus on was giving it what it needed, and sometimes giving it what it desired, liked copious amounts of chocolate and meat pies.

When Cruz was born, however, all the same feelings I had when Oliver arrived came flooding back. I mourned my pregnant body, and hated my post-birth body, this time even worse than before. Whether it was the sleep deprivation or that my body had changed even more, I was in a really crap place. To make things worse, I felt so incredibly guilty for being so self-absorbed, crying on the bathroom floor because my body didn't look like it used to when I was so lucky to have two healthy beautiful babies.

Then my negative self image began to affect those around me, I would often ask Mat to go to social gatherings without me. He never wanted to but I often pleaded with him to go alone as I didn't want to see anyone. I would cry in changing rooms and in bed at night. I would say things to myself that I wouldn't say to my worst enemy.

I felt really alone. I didn't want to talk to friends about how I was feeling because I knew exactly what they would say, 'Taryn you've just had a baby, it's perfectly normal.' So I said nothing, it was just me and the dark passenger inside my head.

One night when Cruz was about six months old, Mat and I went out for dinner and had a couple of drinks. It was the first time in a long time that I had had a couple of drinks (I'm not a drinker, I could go literally months without having one) and I was feeling slightly tipsy. When we got back home, Mat sensed my relaxed mood and before we knew it, it was on. With a couple of drinks under my belt, I didn't care so much about how I looked, and when Mat said to me, 'We aren't using protection, will it be okay?' I said, 'Yes! GO FOR IT, it will be fine.'

A few weeks later, standing in a chicken shop, I couldn't shift a nagging feeling of nausea. Apparently it wasn't fine. Apparently even when you are exclusively breastfeeding, you can still get pregnant – even when it was difficult to conceive the first two children. I raced from the chicken shop straight to the chemist, grabbed a couple of pregnancy tests and sure enough when I peed on the stick, it indicated I was pregnant. I'll never forget the moment I looked at that blue line and said to myself out loud, 'It is going to be a girl, and she is here for a reason.' It's only been in the past couple of years that I've realised the enormity of that moment. Without Mikaela the Body Image Movement wouldn't exist.

So my body image issues were once again disguised by another pregnancy, however this time around I thought proactively about how I would deal with my body loathing after the baby was born. I couldn't do round three in front of the mirror, pulling my stomach fat in disgust, telling myself I was gross. I decided that I was going to get surgery to fix my body after this pregnancy.

It was raining on the day of the surgeon's appointment, and we pulled up in a car park right out the front in Hutt Street, Adelaide. Mat was with me and for good reason. I'm one of these people that doesn't read fine print and if I was ordered to sign my life away that day I would have because I was so excited, so delirious and so ready. Oh so ready. I had been waiting years for this appointment, I had given birth to three children in three and a half years, I had fed over four thousand meals from my breasts and I had suffered prolonged physical pain and emotional distress.

The surgeon's office was very tastefully decorated with amazing artwork of naked females. My foot tapped continuously on the ground as Mat sat next to me twirling the umbrella around and around. Waiting, waiting, waiting, and then...

The surgeon was delightful, but we spent so long (please interpret that to be soooooolooooooong) talking about stuff that really wasn't getting me any closer to slab. He must have picked up on my sense of urgency because finally he said he'd take a look, and I undressed and sat on the table in just my undone jeans. It feels really weird being in a room with a strange man handling your breasts as your husband looks on. Not exactly the threesome you might fantasise about. The surgeon asked me to let my stomach out, I did, and then he said, 'And some more,' and I finally let it go. I look under my brow to see the reaction on Mat's face. My stomach is GIGANTIC, I could pass for a six month pregnant woman. I could have just sank into the carpet I felt so utterly mortified. But wait, there's more.

The surgeon picked up my breasts with his thumbs and index fingers, just like he would do if he was picking up a snot-filled dirty tissue, and tells me there isn't enough breast tissue for me to have just a breast lift, I would need to have implants as well.

He then grabbed my stomach and confirms that he'd get rid of all this (the fat and excess skin) and fix up the boobs and voilà, new body new you! I was so excited, I was like a giddy schoolgirl in love for the first time. The next ten minutes were a bit of a blur, Mat was asking all the sensible questions like, how long the surgery would take, and what were the risks. The only questions I needed answering were, 'What's your diary like?' and, 'When can you schedule my surgery in?'

I almost skipped out of the office, I hadn't felt this validated, excited and energised in months. All the heartache I had been through, the hours spent in agonising in front of the bathroom mirror, all the tears that were shed, all the negative feelings were going to be magically whisked away. My body was going to be fixed.

As we drove away I sensed that Mat was not sharing my jubilation. I always knew he wasn't thrilled about me having major surgery, and if he had a choice in the matter he would have said no. But he wanted to support me, and he wanted me to feel better about my body, so he was quietly doing his best not to burst my bubble.

Going ahead with the surgery meant a lot of family sacrifices would have to be made. All of which I could totally justify because I felt that I was the one who had been sacrificing for years. Sacrificing my self-esteem, sacrificing my body, my sleep – oh the list could go on. Without it sounding like, 'You did this so I am going to do that,' I felt like it was my right to have surgery. I 'deserved' to have it.

Like most couples with a young family we didn't have a lazy $12,000 sitting in the bank account, so we were going to have to borrow the money. Mat was going to have to take a couple of weeks off work, and it was going to have to be all hands on deck when I was in hospital.

The thought of being in hospital and the pain that would follow the surgery didn't bother me one bit, in fact it might be fair to say that as an exhausted mother of three who was up nearly every night to at least one child, the thought of having two weeks in bed, where no one could disturb me, was almost appealing. Not to forget my fondness for hospital sandwiches as previously mentioned.

I spoke to Mum about the surgery and she was as supportive as she could've been. Like Mat she thought it was unnecessary, but would stand by my decision regardless. Telling my friends was much more gratifying. They got it completely, asking all the most important questions like, 'What size boobs are you going to have?'

Nothing was going to stop me from having surgery, I had made up my mind. The logistics of surgery were arranged, all I needed to do was go and have it done. I never expected a change of heart. In fact, you could have knocked me over with a feather. Everything changed in an ordinary moment. As I was watching Mikaela playing on the floor in front of me, I had an epiphany.

The day was just another ordinary day in my crazy house. There were breakfast dishes on the kitchen bench with leftover cereal and excess wasted milk in bowls, there were piles of washing on the floor of the laundry (even though we have a pull out chute for the dirty clothes) and there was probably poop on the back lawn, courtesy of our schnauzer – Ammo.

I was drinking my coffee, watching Mikaela playing with toys on the floor in front of me and thinking about my approaching surgery. I was absolutely convinced that a boob job and a tummy tuck was going to make me happy, and I was wondering just how that would feel, and then out of nowhere it happened. The epiphany.

e·piph·a·ny – *'a sudden, powerful, and often spiritual or life-changing realisation that a person experiences in an otherwise ordinary moment.'*

I'd never experienced an epiphany before but it was like a lightning bolt had come from the sky and hit the ground in front of me when

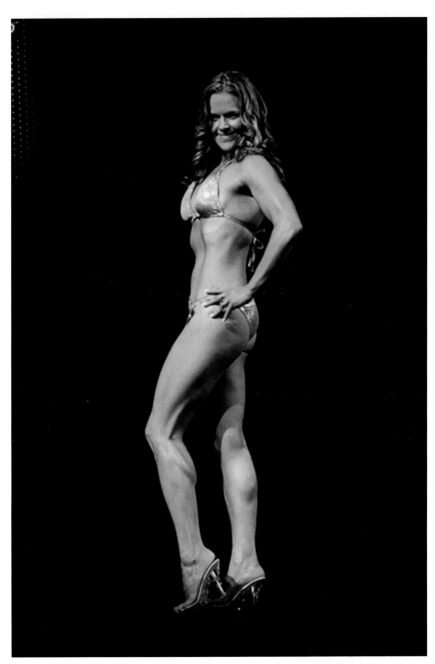

ABOVE: Bright lights, porno shoes and possible camel toe!

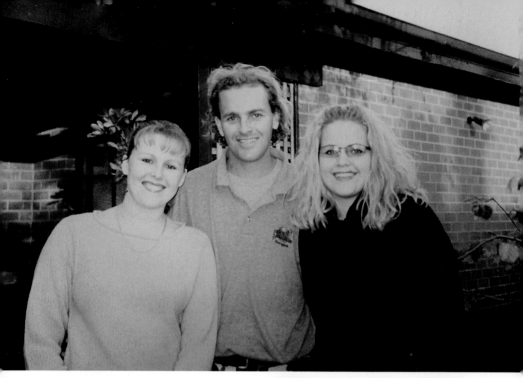

ABOVE: My sister Justine, brother Jason and me on Mother's Day. This was the last time I saw Jason.

RIGHT: Jason and me.

FAR RIGHT ABOVE: One of the only 'grown up' photos I have of my family all together.

FAR RIGHT BELOW: Jason playing Sean Penn's movie double in the film *The Thin Red Line*.

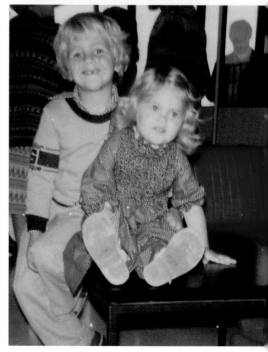

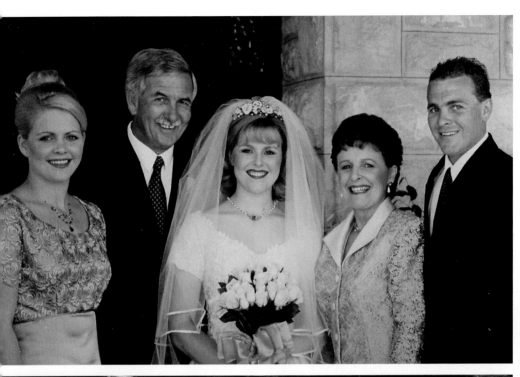

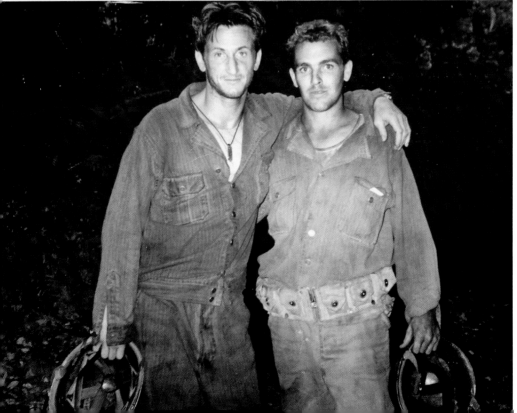

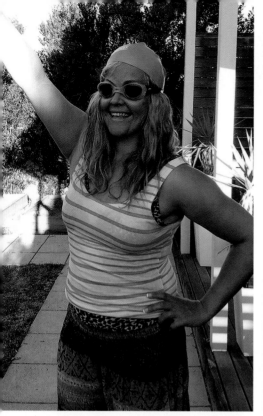

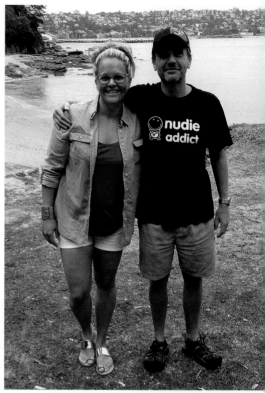

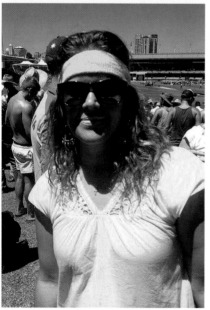

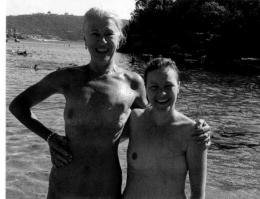

CLOCKWISE FROM TOP LEFT: Training mode for the Sydney Skinny; Nigel Marsh and me at Cobblers Beach on the morning of the Sydney Skinny; two inspiring women from the Sydney Skinny; getting my Australian spirit on at the cricket, the day before I started training for the competition.

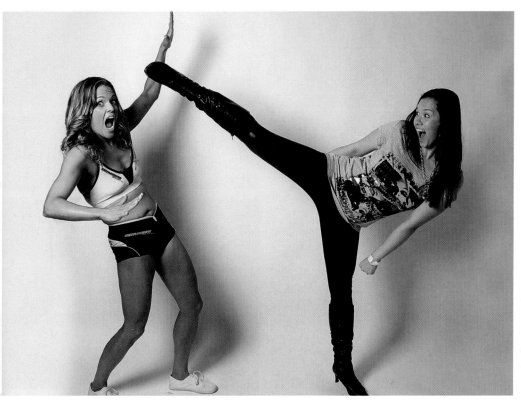

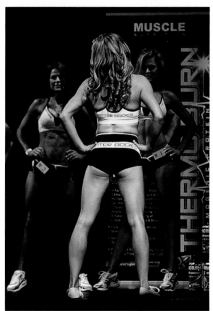

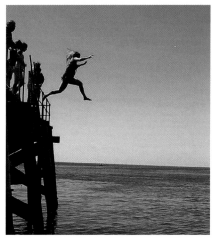

CLOCKWISE FROM TOP LEFT: Taekwondo champion, my trainer and friend Ruth Hock; getting my sparkle on, jetty-jumping style; please note how high I've pulled these guys up, yep Harry Highpanting big time.

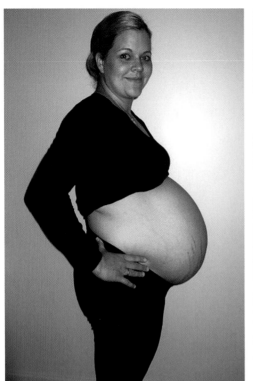
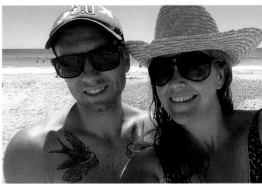
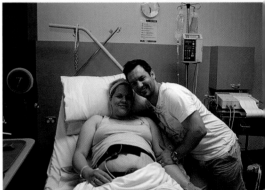
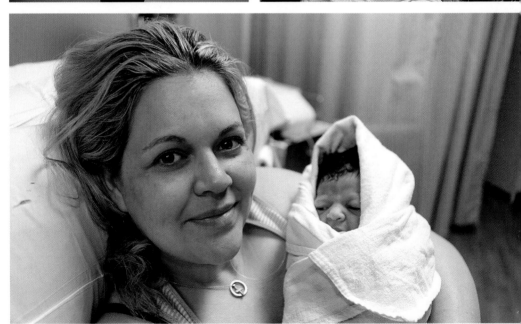

CLOCKWISE FROM TOP LEFT: 38 weeks pregnant with Oliver; Mat and I hanging at one of our favourite places – Willunga Beach, Adelaide; becoming a Mum and Dad; ah 'that' moment, there is nothing more joyous than holding your new baby.

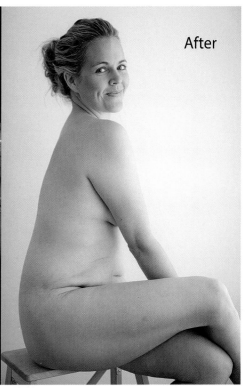

Before

After

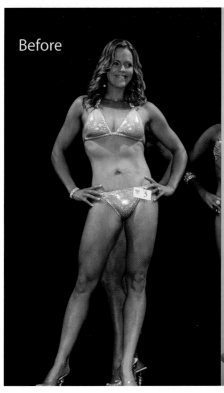

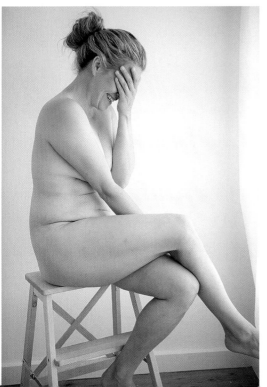

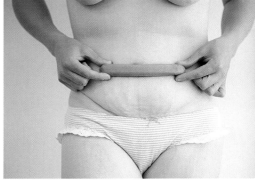

CLOCKWISE FROM TOP: The before and after photo; that photo ... let's never mention this again; 'that moment' in a photoshoot when the postman rides slowly past the window!

OVERLEAF: The 're-enactment' of the 'nipples the size of dinner plates'.

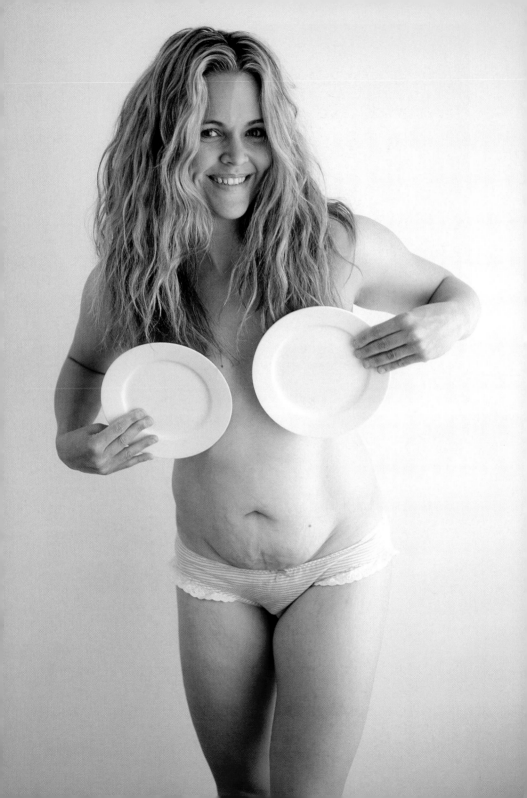

this thought struck me: How am I going to teach Mikaela to love her body if I can't do the same? Followed by an onslaught of more questions coming at me, thick and fast and unrelenting...

- How am I ever going to encourage her to accept and love the parts of her body that she doesn't like without being a walking contradiction?

- If I go ahead with the surgery am I setting my daughter up for a future of body hatred and self-loathing?

- In ten years time when she becomes a teenager will she want to be like her mummy and have manufactured breasts and a surgically produced flat stomach?

- Am I setting her up to chase an unrealistic goal of perfection?

- Will she place more value on her looks than what she achieves in life because her mummy has placed so much emphasis on her own 'beauty'?

Oh! The guilt and the shame I experienced right there in that moment, when I thought to myself, 'Taryn you are a mother now, you can't make decisions based only on your own needs, you have your babies to consider.'

Like most mothers I want to protect and love my children. If I had to make a choice over their welfare or my own, there is no decision to make, they are always priority number one. I remember growing up and watching movies and when there was a life or death situation for a parent and a child, the parent would always put the child first. I always wondered about this, I used to question it: 'Seriously, would they REALLY give up their life for their child?' But I get it now, there is no love like the love you have for your child. I remember the birth of each of our children and that feeling of holding them for the first time. For me, it was instant love. In that very moment of looking at them for the first time, I would die for them, I would do anything for them.

It never occurred to me until that moment that my boob job and tummy tuck would potentially affect the relationship that Mikaela has with her body as she gets older.

I didn't want to put her in that position. I didn't want to be the reason that she hated her body, or the reason that she wanted to change her body. I couldn't bear to be a walking talking contradiction either, attempting to teach her to love her body if I couldn't embrace mine. I had to be a positive role model for her. Going ahead with the surgery was not going to be the best decision for Miki.

If you are reading this and have children and did have surgery – please don't think I'm suggesting that those who have had surgery are bad role models for their children. These were my decisions, this is my unique story and everyone has their own life story. What I am saying is that there is no room for guilt, it's a wasted emotion, and after all we are just doing the best we can do.

Who knew that after that day my life would change so dramatically and take a turn in a completely different direction? Life is so unpredictable.

I spent the next few days feeling really despondent. I just knew I wasn't going to be able to go through with the surgery but the thought of living with my existing body threw me into despair. This is when I hit rock bottom. I felt completely trapped, I so desperately wanted to fix my body but my hands were tied. For days I moped around the house, I cried, I even headed back to standing in front of the mirror giving myself a hard time. And then I thought to myself, 'Fuckin' hell Taryn, this is ridiculous, you can't live like this for the rest of your life.'

I decided to speak to Mat about the epiphany. As soon as I said the word 'epiphany' I knew he just wanted to roll his eyes. Mat and I are like chalk and cheese, and the older we get the more differently we operate, but somehow it seems to work for us. Mat is methodical and strategic in his approach when making decisions, while I operate on intuition and 'putting things out to the universe'. Once we'd got past the epiphany word and I started saying things like, 'I don't think I can go ahead with the surgery because I'm worried how it will affect Mikaela when she is older,' I had his full attention. He got it, he understood where I was coming from, and he respected my decision.

Making the phone call to the surgeon's office to say that I would no longer be requiring his services was tough. It took all my willpower to speak the words, 'I need to cancel my appointment, I no longer need the surgery.' I couldn't tell the surgeon I didn't 'want' it anymore, because it wasn't true. I hung up the phone, and that's when I lost it, I sat on the ground looking at the cordless phone in my hand with tears running down my face.

The reality of what I was doing was sinking in. I don't want to go back to a living hell of hating my body. Would I ever be able to get back to the person I used to be? Would I remain a recluse forever? How would I be able to continue this Oscar award-winning performance convincing my close friends and family that I was happy and content without a social life.

Where do I go from here?

CHAPTER SIX

Turning it all around

ALBERT EINSTEIN ONCE DEFINED INSANITY AS doing the same thing over and over again and expecting different results. I had made my decision not to have the surgery, and I was sticking with that, so my choices moving forward were very clear. I could either spend the rest of my life wanting to change my body but doing nothing about it, or I could make positive decisions in my life that would alter the parts of my body I had control over.

One day when I was feeling frustrated with the dark passenger's unrelenting voice inside my head, I grabbed a piece of paper and drew a line down the middle, on one side I wrote 'change' and on the other I wrote 'accept'.

I had a conversation with myself, 'Right Taryn, the shape of your boobs, the fact that you've had babies, and the stretch marks are here to stay, so are you going to fight for changes that aren't going to happen or are you going to accept them for what they are?' I then wrote on the Accept side: boobs, stretch marks.

'And what are things about your body that you could change that would positively impact your life, health or happiness? 'I then wrote on the Change side: nails (I am the world's most committed nail biter), fitness and bags under the eyes.

Change	Accept
Nails	Boob shape
Fitness	Stretch marks
Bags under the eyes	Childbearing tummy

From that first day until now my brain works on an entirely different operating system. I've taken the power away from the dark passenger and I work on a fact-based approach to problem-solving my body woes. It didn't mean that 'ugly' thoughts would no longer pop into my head, it just meant that when they did I wasn't 'buying in' to the bullshit and feeding the problem. Oh, and there was a lot of faking it until I made it in those early days.

I didn't wake up one day and LOVE looking at myself in the mirror. But rather than rubbishing the crap out of myself I would just not say anything at all. Eventually over time I was able to say something nice to myself and before you know it, a monster of positivity was born, and in front of the mirror I would say things like, 'You hawwwwt minx you, you sexy mamma, how are you going to fend back the men today? Nah, just kidding, I never said anything like that but I definitely stopped saying things like, 'You are fat, ugly and disgusting,' that's for sure.

Without realising it at the time, I was on an unplanned and unconscious self-help experimental journey, and it worked. The strategies that I implemented in those early days, as simple as they were, changed my life and have since changed thousands of lives since. And the best thing about it was it didn't cost $12,000!

In those early days, however, I was still a rookie in the world of body lovin' and certainly no expert! I was also very afraid of relapsing and often asked myself whether I had 'tricked' myself into loving my body – did I love it or was I faking it? It wasn't until I implemented the SUCK IT UP strategy that I really felt strong, and the love for my body became one hundred per cent unbreakable.

Ever since I was a small child I have always felt considerable emotion for others who are suffering. It's a trait I see in my beautiful eldest son Oliver who has a level of empathy beyond his years. This is a really bad example but it is delightfully beautiful at the same time. A few months ago, Oliver and I were watching an Austin Powers movie, it was the scene when Dr. Evil finds out that Sir Nigel Powers is his dad. The scene is ridiculously funny and over the top, and when Dr. Evil and his dad connect and embrace, I hear a little snuffle coming from the little human sitting next to me. Oliver was in tears. It was in that moment I just knew that Oliver had the same compassion and empathy as I did for others. I just knew he felt what I so often feel, above and beyond what most people feel – I think.

I remembered one of the first times I felt empathy was at primary school. The first thing I wrote about in Year 1 at school was the starving Ethiopian children.

'Ethiopia Ethiopia the poor children of Ethiopia

Ethiopia Ethiopia the children are starving in Ethiopia

Ethiopia Ethiopia we must help the children of Ethiopia'

Then I drew a hut, with a sign that said '10,000 people live in here'.

Even as I write this now I have tears in my eyes, those words were the first sentence I remember writing as a child and the emotion attached to them have stayed with me. I am not sure what I saw, or who I spoke to from the age of nought to five, but someone or something had a profound effect on me. To think that there are people in the world who can't access food and water breaks my heart. It was these thoughts that led me to another technique that I use to help me overcome my body image issues, the technique I called 'hovering'.

Hovering is an exercise in gratitude and perspective, something I think is lacking in a lot of people, and is when you take some quiet time to reflect on how others live in the world. Pretend you are hovering above the earth and looking down at different countries and different cultures, in particular, look at how other women are living their lives.

The technique came to be on a day that I was having a particularly self-indulgent moment. I was trying to find a nice top to wear and nothing was looking right: too tight, too loose, too fat, too ugly. I was pining for a nice perky set of boobs and felt annoyed that I had a set of teabags instead. I went and grabbed a cuppa and sat on the couch and was reflecting on my woes, when I remembered my Change and Accept list and mentally re-popped the boobs on the accept side and thought, 'Seriously Taryn, get on with it, you are so lucky to have what you have, you are being a brat.' As I sat there in my lovely house, with my designer white walls, drinking my skinny latte my mind drifted off to what other people might be doing in that exact moment in different parts of the world. I wasn't thinking of all the nice things, I was thinking of the hardship, pain and sadness.

I thought about a land of war and famine. I imagined a mother holding her dying child. I could see the child's eyes in my mind, big, brown and hopeful. I felt the despair and hopelessness of the mother, unable to give what her child what she needed to live. In my mind like watching a film, I saw the baby die and I could hear the screams of the mother. I watched as the mother held her lifeless child, kissing her cheeks, her forehead, holding her tight. She was sobbing.

There were tears running down my face. I felt the pain. While the visions in my head were just made up, the stories of a grieving woman and a child dying of hunger were very real. Every few seconds a child dies and a mother's spirit is broken.

And here I am, unable to decide on something to wear, feeling sorry for myself.

I continued hovering above the world, imagining the lives of other people less fortunate than me. I came to India. There was a 12-year-old who had been kidnapped from her home and trafficked to another town, an hour from her house. She was alone and petrified sitting in an empty room with just a bed and a dirty sheet on top. Men came into the room, one by one looking at her and leaving. Outside, her virginity was being auctioned off.

And here I am, upset because I can't find a top that fits me right?

That day on the couch I took myself all around the world in ways I'd never travelled. I knew from that moment on I had a duty to those less fortunate than me, I had a responsibility to live my life with respect and gratitude.

Hovering for me was inspiring and it snapped me out of my self-indulgence. How could I bang on about such trivial matters when the world around me was filled with atrocities and sadness.

This practical exercise on gratitude then turned into the 'Suck it up' concept.

The more I worked on Suck it up, the happier I became. I not only applied Suck it up to my body image challenges, I applied it to all aspects of life. It was as if a weight was lifted from my shoulders, I really didn't have a care in the world, in fact, nothing REALLY mattered – except all the important stuff.

Having allowed myself to step outside of my bubble of a life and walk in the shoes of others, it made me stop and reflect how good I had it. What a beautiful blessed existence I was living! Sure I've been challenged over the years with the bullying, tragic deaths of loved ones and body image issues but really, in the context of the world we live in, I am nothing short of extremely lucky.

I decided to blog about Suck it up, because it had been such a powerful strategy for me to use on my journey of body acceptance. Some people took great exception to it though; here's what some of them had to say:

'Being told to 'suck it up' is an appalling message to send to women who are probably already suffering from shame and low self worth.'

'Suck it up is one big dismissal of 'first world problems'. It serves only to shame women for what are, to some, real and debilitating problems.'

'I don't agree our problems are lesser because someone has it worse.'

'Grossly oversimplifying people's problems because you deem them not important enough to worry about is not the answer!'

Well, it was the answer for me, or just one of the answers anyway.

Reading some of the comments that people had made in response to my article on made me feel a little sad. I adore people and it would never be my intention to offend or shame ANYONE. I certainly wouldn't tell someone with an eating disorder or someone dealing with depression to 'suck it up'. That just wouldn't be cool. But I'm sure there are a vast number of people who could really benefit from being told to stop carrying on like pork chops once in a while. People's whose dialogue is, 'I wish I didn't have...' 'I want more of...' 'She's so lucky she's got...' 'I hate my...'

We live in a beauty-obsessed society, and part of the reason is because we've been preyed upon and reprogrammed by the diet and beauty industry to want to be something other than what we are. On a constant basis we are being told to change, to look different, to defy something, to lose something and to compare ourselves to people who are declared to be more attractive and therefore more successful and more powerful. The emphasis on beauty seems to take a greater priority in people's lives than their health.

I know it did in mine. And yet if someone sat me down and asked me, 'What is more important, your health or your beauty?' I am sure I would have said health, it's just that my actions hadn't supported that. Back in the days of self-loathing I was so consumed by how I looked. I would preen, prune, strip, clip, burn, lose, rub and defy anything and everything I could about my body. Beauty was the currency and my health took a back seat. It just didn't sit with me, so after I implemented the Change and Accept list, followed by Suck it up, the third thing I did was begin focusing on putting my health before beauty. This was the time that I recognised that my body was not an ornament but rather a vehicle to my dreams.

Instead of running to lose weight, I started to run because I loved being outdoors and I loved the feeling of accomplishment that running gave me. Instead of going to the gym to tighten up, I went to the gym because I loved boxing with my girlfriends and sweating up a storm. Instead of restricting what I ate for weight loss, I would eat to fuel my body.

Eating and physical exercise took on a whole new meaning. I felt so good, I was oozing energy and happiness. I found it near impossible to be down about my body, because the endorphins were flowing.

During this time of 'self exploration' there was no grand plan, there was no thought of the Body Image Movement, it was just me doing what I could do to enjoy life and stop hating my body. And I achieved just that. I didn't loathe my body like I used to, but even after months and months of positive affirmations and feeling good, there was one question that continued to pop up in my head, over and over.

What does it feel like to have the perfect body?

CHAPTER SEVEN

Fitness competition

THE BEST THING ABOUT SATURDAY MORNINGS was heading to the gym to do Ruth's boxing class, which I'd carried on taking, on and off, between pregnancies. Ruth was hardcore, she didn't mince her words and I liked her style. Truth be told, I thought that she'd make a good friend. I am not a fan of smoke and mirrors when it comes to friendships, I always like to know where I stand. If I've made a mistake or acted like a knob then a good, confident friend would tell me so; I like confident women and Ruth was definitely that.

It is probably also fair to say that, embarrassingly, I wanted to impress Ruth with my boxing style and my commitment to being the fastest and the hardest. I knew that Ruth had been a Taekwondo world champion, so I hoped she would see the Rocky Balboa in me. And sure enough she did, right after I extended the friendship branch by bringing in some of Mikaela's old baby clothes. It was a nice ice breaker and the perfect opportunity for me to tell her I used to eat raw eggs for breakfast and run up stairs with my hoody on.

For weeks the other girls in the class and I speculated about Ruth's growing tummy, but she said nothing and kicked and punched with no reservation or hesitation. And then one day it was blaringly obvious. I was slightly devastated when I found out Ruth was pregnant, I was going to lose my favourite (ever) gym instructor and my blissful Saturday mornings were never going to be the same.

During one of my conversations with Ruth I mentioned I was a photographer, and she wanted some bump photos taken, so I thought here is my opportunity. Rather than charging Ruth a fee, I would do a contra-deal that she carry on working with me as a personal trainer, after her boxing classes finished.

Weekly personal training sessions were tough, but fun and rewarding too. It was easy for me to train at the gym because the gym had a crèche and all three kids enjoyed being there with Sue the Crèche Manager and her delightful staff. There was a two-hour crèche limit, which was plenty of time to do a session then head into the sauna for twenty minutes before a relaxing long hot shower. I had found my groove and I was really enjoying working out.

Then came the day when I told Ruth I couldn't get the thought of how it would feel to have the perfect body out of my head. Ruth had heard me rant endlessly about body image, and how I was feeling and what I was thinking, but this question was new. In typical nonchalant Ruth style, in her Canadian accent, she said, 'Well why don't you enter a fitness model competition?' I scoffed at her, 'You are kidding me, right? I can't do that. I am a mother of three, with THIS stomach, I cannot stand up on a stage in front of hundreds of people and I've not worn a bikini well since, well... never actually.'

I'm not sure if it was the way she looked at me or the words 'I can't' echoing around my brain, but by the time we'd talked about it a bit more, and she had explained why she thought it wasn't a completely insane idea, I walked out of the gym that day heading home to start some online research and do some serious thinking.

By the time Mat arrived home that evening I was just BUSTING to talk to him about my plans. Ruth had done a competition herself just the year before and had insisted that I sit down with Mat and have a big chat about the time and money commitment, and the impact it would have on my family. When I told Mat about it, his initial reaction was, you've guessed it, eye roll, followed by, 'Here we go again, another one of your bright ideas.' In his defence, I have come home with a few 'Best Ever' plans over the years. Things like,

'We are going to raise $5,000 for a cancer charity by standing at the train station with forty of our friends, all dressed as super heroes!' (we did, ending up with $7,000 but standing for twelve hours when eight months pregnant was less than ideal), and then there was the time I decided to record a song, and the time I set up my photography business having owned a camera for less than three months. So, Mat had admittedly seen many ideas come through our doors, but this one was a little different.

Knowing me so well, and how much I love food, he doubted that I could follow the restrictions on how much, and what, a fitness model eats. He didn't want to discourage me but he had to be honest, he didn't think I had the discipline to follow a regimented food diet. Ever since Mat and I got together my weight had been up and down like a yoyo. I would eat too much crap, I'd put weight on, I'd sign up to Weight Watchers, I'd lose weight and then I'd repeat the cycle again. We often joked that I was a WWW, (Weight Watchers Whore), I would always be going back for more and more.

I decided that evening I was going to enter the competition. But first things first, I had to enjoy as many meals and as much chocolate as I could. Chocolate is my thing. I am not a fan of wine, so at the end of a long day, instead of a glass of wine I would grab a block of chocolate. How was I going to get through fifteen weeks without my favourite treat?

When Ruth emailed me through my eating plan I was sooooo pumped. If you are a yoyo dieter like me, you'll appreciate the excitement and the hope that starting a new regime brings. Whether it was the Atkins diet, the combination diet or one of those twelve-week transformation programs, getting a 'what you can eat list' is as exciting for me as squeezing a pimple or plucking my eyebrows (yes, I find it therapeutic).

As I sat down to prepare my menus and begin writing shopping lists for the array of food I was going to be eating, something struck me as odd. Where is all the food on the list? Why am I eating all the same foods every day? Why is there so much chicken? And as I don't eat vegetables, why has broccoli made it on here?

It become apparent that some food negotiation was in order. Here's how the conversation went:

Me: 'Hey Ruth, this meal plan sucks, I definitely can't eat vegetables, I hate vegetables.'

Ruth: 'Well, you are just going to have to get used to them.'

Me: 'Ruth, my mother already tried that for about fifteen years, if you think I'm going to be eating veggies in the next fifteen weeks it's not going to happen!'

Ruth: 'Taryn.' I sink a little lower, she never calls me by my name like that. 'Taryn, the competition is tough, the girls you will be standing on stage with will have been training for months, years even, you are going to have to stick to the diet, no ifs or buts. You need to be one hundred per cent committed. No exceptions.'

Far out, I loved Ruth to bits, she was merciless. Eventually, however, my polite persistence wore down her resistance and after weeks of nagging I was able to substitute some vegetables for salad, and at around week three when I continued to gag on tuna I was able to substitute it with salmon.

One of the hardest meal times was going out with friends for dinner. I remember one night, very early in the program, going to a Thai restaurant. Everyone was tucking into the most amazing banquet while I ate boiled chicken, plain rice and greens. These were the hardest and most testing moments. Fish and chips at the beach sans the fish and the chips was challenging too. Watching the kids crunching the chips in between their teeth and just the mere thought of chicken salt made my mouth salivate. I missed food, I mourned it every single day. But fifteen weeks of eating almost 'to the letter' was a real triumph for me, I was in fact really proud of sticking to it, pushing through the pain and exercising control and discipline – something that I've been known in the past not to execute too well. I've always approached diets truly believing that I will do the right thing, only to find myself a few days in saying, 'Oh fuck it, life is short, I might die tomorrow, I am so having that slice of pizza!'

The saving grace in my week's line up of boring meals was my cheat meal. For one meal a week I could have whatever I wanted, with a glass of wine. (Of course I substituted the wine for some chocolate.) The way I ate cheat meals was like holding back an orgasm, I didn't want to eat too fast, I wanted to savour every single mouthful and I definitely never wanted it to end.

I can understand why so many girls who train to do fitness model and bodybuilding competitions develop eating disorders. Everything about my fixation with food was disordered. When I wasn't thinking about or craving food, I was weighing food, and when I wasn't weighing food I was preparing food. Food, food, food, it has always been something I focus on, but this was definitely the most obsessed I'd been in my entire life.

As tough as the diet was, there was another component of the program that was equally challenging – the physical training. My training schedule looked like this:

Mondays: Quads, calves and abs (pfft, abs what were they?!).

Tuesday: Back, shoulders and biceps.

Wednesday: Glutes, hamstrings and abs (pfft, you can put them in twice a week but they are still M.I.A.).

Friday: Chest and triceps.

Now that looks pretty reasonable when you look at it written down like that, but on top of the weight sessions I was at the gym six days a week to do my cardio on an empty stomach. That meant that every morning except Sunday I was up at 5.30am and working out at 6am for at least one hour. It was really hard, especially as I am NOT a morning person!

Within just a few weeks, however, I noticed the weight was coming off, and I saw muscles developing in parts of my body that I'd never seen one before. Everyone around me started noticing that I was up to something and eventually I told people. Most of their reactions were, 'YOU'RE DOING WHAT??!!!' I didn't tell most of my friends until about half-way into the training. I'm not a fan of people that are 'gonnas', I'm gonna to do this and I'm gonna to do that. I'd rather say nothing and just do it. It took me at least six weeks to actually believe that I would achieve what I'd set out to do, telling people any earlier would've put too much pressure on.

During week eight of the fifteen-week training schedule, Ruth presented me with another training and diet plan. Here's how that dialogue went:

Me: 'What's this?'

Ruth: 'Your new schedule.'

Me: 'Why? What's wrong with the one I've got?'

Ruth: 'It's time to ramp things up.'

Me: 'WHAT THE...? Surely things can't get harder, or more restrictive? Can they? What is it exactly that you want me to ramp up? I am giving you all I've got.'

Ruth: 'Then you'll have to find some more!'

The truth is, I did have more in the tank. We humans have two very powerful primal instincts, one is to avoid pain and the other is to move towards pleasure. I was merely acting like any normal human being for those first eight weeks, just leaving a little in the tank. Ruth was right, she always was, I needed to up the ante.

So I did – training six days a week, doing cardio for at least one and a half hours but more often two hours a day. More days than not I trained twice. It was all-consuming and as much as I tried to protect my little ones from the rigour of my routine, it was impossible for anyone around me not to be affected.

Mat and I would often fight, I was, after all, so hideously grumpy. I couldn't count on all my fingers and toes the amount of times he yelled, 'Just go and eat something, would you!' Then of course there was the toll it took on my children, I was never there when they woke up in the morning and I was often too distracted by thoughts of my body or the competition to be a fully 'present' mother. Living mindfully is something that I strive to do, but during training, unless I was at the gym, I was very removed from the present moment.

There was a lot of sacrifice from us all in those fifteen weeks of training that no one really knew about. Most people just saw the end result of a transformed body, but didn't realise the personal and family sacrifice needed to achieve it. Even trivial things like having to wash my very thick and long hair every day grated on me. Washing and combing my hair takes about thirty minutes, that's three and a half hours a week! It doesn't sound like much, but when your workouts are already eating up three hours of your day, it is!

So, I've filled you in on the journey to that stage and the weeks in which I forced my body into a particular shape, and how at the end of the process I stood in front of an audience of seven hundred, being judged on how well I'd done. The second round of the competition (after bikini) was sportswear. It was so going to be my time to shine, wearing clothes and a sensible pair of flat running shoes instead of porno shoes – I was ready to smash my walk out the park! Of course that was just my ego speaking because, get me out there, for round two I was still shitting myself! The lights were still bright, I could still see my dad's silver fox hair and I could definitely hear my friends screaming. Round One was just a warm up for my entourage, they really got into it in the second round.

I didn't win any prize or even get placed, but actually, after all that, for once in my life it wasn't about winning, it was about not falling over when I walked on stage, and not looking like a twat. I was the oldest contestant and there wasn't anyone up there that had given birth to three kids, again, just pointing that out – okay?!

Stepping off stage I'd never felt more relieved – I had done it, I had taken complete control over my body and perfected it into something that I had thought wasn't possible, and I had paraded half naked in front of a crown of strangers, without dropping my smile. I never thought I could, but it went off without a hitch. I couldn't wait to go out for dinner and eat! And eat I did. I remember sitting at the restaurant with my folks, Kelley and a handful of friends just drooling over the menu. I remember thinking on this night and for weeks to come, 'I can eat anything I want! ANYTHING!' It was such a liberating and exciting feeling!

The next day was Mother's Day and after a sleep in, it was time to indulge my appetite big time! I'd been warned not to go 'too crazy' after being on such a restrictive diet, but seriously are you kidding me, I will be eating everything in sight and no one can stop me! Eggs Benedict with extra Hollandaise for breakfast, juice, coffee and a handful of chocolate eggs. Being a chocolate addict and not being able to eat Easter eggs over Easter had been torture! I had some making up to do!

Competing changed me. It helped me to realise that I could achieve anything I wanted to. It taught me to never say never. There were so many times I could've walked away but I didn't. I stuck to it, and showed more determination and discipline than I ever had before.

CHAPTER EIGHT

Who do you think you are?

APART FROM COMMENTS LIKE, 'You've got your hands full,' and, 'You should speak with Dove,' the other line I hear often is, 'I don't know how you do it!', and my own often repeated question, 'Who do I think I am?' asking whether I really think I'm up to the job. And you know what, there have been plenty of times when I've thrown my hands up in the air and thought to myself 'I DON'T know how I do it!'

During my time working in New Zealand as Operations Manager for an international hotel marketing company, I was always trying to be harder, stronger, wiser, more infallible than anyone else. I'm not sure whether it was because I was in a boys' club (female managers were few and far between) but at all times I followed one strict rule, 'Always look like you know what you are doing.'

One day, however, I became unstuck, and it was very public and it was highly embarrassing. We were in Singapore for a work conference and over one hundred managers from all over the world had flown in. This was a time when multinational companies had trucks of money to splash around on teambuilding events for their employees, so not only had we spent a few days on a cruise liner, we'd also been through the streets of Singapore on rickshaws, boats and cars following an *Amazing Race* style 'treasure hunt'. The conference was drawing to a close, and each region's Operations Managers had to present their sales strategy and forecast for the following year. There were two Ops Managers in my region – me and Mark. I seriously did not want to be the one to do the presentation. I went to the bathroom to get myself together but the nerves had already taken over – my stomach was filled with butterflies and my breathing had turned very shallow. It wasn't that I didn't know the information, I could have provided that with my eyes closed, it was presenting it to front of a room of people that had me in a tailspin.

Mark and I spent a few hours putting together our presentation and then it was time to deliver it. Because of my fear of public speaking, the plan was that Mark would present and that at three points I would give short one sentence examples to support what he was saying.

Because all the other regions had gone before us and we were (unsurprisingly) the last, I'd been able to watch their presentations, and had noticed that each of them had taken the opportunity to speak. After all, if you are ever going to climb the corporate ladder, this was the perfect opportunity – a room filled with senior management was THE time to impress. I could see there was often a battle for airtime, with the managers – usually men – trying to outdo each other, using buzzwords and jargon such as 'synergy', 'paradigm shifts', and 'globalisation'.

We stood up in front of everyone, Mark did his thing, and like the pretty female assistant to a game show host I played supporting role. I stood next to Mark, with nothing to say, while he talked for up to ten minutes at time. Can you imagine what that looked like? Me standing there like an ornament, with an increasingly strained interested/involved look on my face, occasionally nodding in an attempt to seem like part of the presentation. It was very clear that I was not. I felt very sidelined and incredibly embarrassed. For years I had worked hard to prove I knew what I was doing, and the gig was finally up, my flaws were on show for everyone to see.

Later that evening, the guys were at the bar drinking, I had one drink and decided to call it a night. I said goodnight to everyone and as I was walking away one of the managers yelled across the floor (in front of everyone), 'Hey Taryn, leave the door ajar!' It took me a moment to grasp what he was saying, basically he was inferring that he was coming up my room later on. I laughed it off as if it were joke. I thought to myself if Mat had been here he would've given him a hiding for being so disrespectful, but by the time I got to my room the tears had welled up in my eyes. Had I lost the respect of my colleagues (after spending years to gain it) because I made myself look like a hostess from *The Wheel of Fortune*?

This experience taught me a valuable lesson and helped build a foundation for my resolve in starting up The Body Image Movement.

After I completed the competition I felt compelled to share what I had learnt over the past twelve months, so I started the Body Image Campaign on Facebook. I posted my first update in July of 2012 with a sad photo of me with the caption 'There was once a place so dark and so sad that no one knew existed'. It got sixteen likes.

This world of body image was new territory for me, I was definitely no expert and I was reminded of this fact many times by the pack of wolves that circled me waiting for me to make a mistake. There was one local woman in particular who gave me a really hard time, often posting lengthy derogatory comments about my opinions. I think she took pleasure in trying to publicly shred me. She was the typical keyboard warrior sitting behind her desk in her self-appointed 'fat activist' role.

As much as I tried to ignore her, she threw me, and for a few months she had me on edge. I spent hours and hours researching and studying to get myself up to speed, so I would look like I knew what I was doing. After all I was talking big. Take a look at one of my posts from just a few months after I started the 'campaign':

'Hey all, don't forget to 'like' the page to keep up with the news, info on the Body Image launch and how you can support and shape the future of our world for the next generation...'

It wasn't that I was being dishonest or peddling bullshit when I used phrases such as 'shape the future of our world for the next generation,' I absolutely believed that was what I wanted to do, I just didn't know how I was going to do it.

A few months into the campaign I changed the name from the Body Image Campaign to Body Image Movement (BIM), and engaged a designer to create a logo for me. Once that was sorted, I did what anyone with more passion than common sense would probably do and went out and spent a small fortune on getting Body Image Movement t-shirts, hats and other random bits of paraphernalia made, and collaborated with others to write an e-book. Yes, I was going to spread my message far and wide by being a walking talking advertisement for positive body image.

I made many mistakes in those early days. The biggest was sharing my negative opinions on other women who I thought had got it wrong, and the small but vocal BIM following made it clear that's not what they wanted to hear from me. One example of this was when I posted a blog about a woman in America who was on a reality TV show called *Plastic Wives*, which follows the lives and cosmetic procedures of a group of plastic surgeons' spouses. This particular woman, who admits to visiting the clinic on almost a daily basis, produced on the show a plastic jar containing a fleshy orange blob suspended in pickling juice. It was, she announced, her labia, 'I think she looks better in the jar,' she said nonchalantly, 'Than hanging down there.' She had had a labia reduction.

In my blog I wrote:

'Now most of you who read my blogs or follow me on Facebook and Twitter know that I really do my best to not make judgements of others' decisions. BUT, on this occasion I have to be nothing but brutally honest, because there is a freaking labia in that woman's jar, (and not for any valid medical reason) So, time out; I'm 'paused' from my niceness for this blog. Because... This woman is a bloody fool.

Eek, even as I wrote that, I felt a pang of guilt, maybe I might tone it down, ready... um, this woman's decision is really, really... SILLY!'

There were mixed comments in response to this, some people wholeheartedly agreed with my opinion while others were 'disappointed' (ouch) in the way I judged her choices. It was my first real Body Image Movement mistake, and it didn't feel good. All I wanted to do was to respond to those people who disapproved of my decision to write the blog in the way that I did with facts and statistics that made my views relevant, credible and justified. I had desperately wanted 'to look like I knew what I was doing'. It took me a day to get my head around how I felt, and I realised I had written the wrong response, it wasn't appropriate to be so harsh on this woman. I hadn't walked in her shoes, who knows what underlying insecurities or experiences in her life had led her to believe her labia needed to be smaller?

So, with my tail between my legs, the next day I posted an apology:

'Re BLOG: Is that really a part of your vagina in that jar?

I made a mistake. I was wrong to judge. I didn't feel good when I was writing the blog, in fact every time I looked at the woman's photo I wondered about her life story, (and what led her to the decisions she made). If I hadn't had my moment of clarity (the epiphany) I might've had surgery and it would've been no one's business to judge me. So a great (public) lesson for me to learn. And from here on in, I will continue to be the non-judging and positive person that I am.

Big love to all far and wide! And thanks to those that helped me see what I already knew.'

The minute I posted this I felt a weight lift off my shoulders. I had finally realised that I don't always have to look like I know what I am doing, I can just 'be me' and everything else will fall into place. I decided that there were no wrong answers when you speak the truth and when you speak from the heart. I could make mistakes and things would still be okay.

Another time I made comments about a woman's choices and the media lapped it up, was about a year after the fitness competition – when I, along with many other people, took great exception to Maria Kang's, 'What's your excuse?' photograph, posted on Facebook.

Maria Kang lives in L.A. where she runs a fitness-focused non-profit organisation, and the photograph she posted shows her in a workout bra and micro shorts revealing her post-baby toned body, kneeling beside her three children, with the caption 'What's your excuse?' and a link to her website. Sheesh, did she come under fire for posting this photo. Women all over the world were offended by what they interpreted as her insensitive and judgemental approach, and they sure let her know about it with tens of thousands of angry Facebook comments.

Here's what I think about it. Posting a picture of yourself with a six-pack and your children (and noting their ages) reeks of condescension. I think it makes many women feel inadequate about their own bodies and their lifestyle choices. Maria's intention was to motivate people to create positive change in their life, but I think she went about it the wrong way. Time and time again research suggests that motivation through emotions of guilt, negativity or fear does not work long term.

I think Maria's photo succeeds in motivating a small minority but for the rest of us doesn't impact positively at all.

I responded to Maria's photo via a blog on Australia's most popular women's website, Mamamia, and within hours it had thousands of shares. Before I knew it I was pegged as Maria's arch enemy and was being interviewed on *Good Morning America* and other outlets across the United States, as well as a handful of TV channels in Australia. It was interesting to see how the media played me against Maria, I even had a local TV show come to my house in Adelaide and ask me to comment 'in a particular way' about Maria. They were actually quite specific about the words, and even the tone (angry), that they wanted me to use. Um, NO! I cannot and will not! I couldn't believe that I was being asked to be nasty to this woman. They wanted a cat fight, but I was determined not to give it to them.

In response I said in my blog that for most of us to have a body like Maria's it would take hours of strength conditioning, a strict diet and a whole lot of time spent exercising. When I say exercising I don't mean a casual walk around the block, or a ride to the beach on your bike, I mean a serious and intensive workout, on a daily basis. For most of us who enjoy a balanced life, if you want to look like Maria, unless you have the genetic disposition that supports that body type, having the near 'perfect' body will take a lot of time, sweat and tears.

I didn't like Maria's photo, I didn't like what the title implied, but that didn't mean I didn't like her. So I decided to contact her, I emailed her and explained my side of the argument. This is what I wrote:

'If you're able to Skype, I'd love the opportunity to chat, and see if we can turn this debate into a positive one for women. I truly believe we both come from the same place. Most of the feedback I am reading is negative about women 'slaggin' each other (which is a real shame because I certainly didn't slag you off, my opinion is just different to yours).

I am wondering if there is something that we could do (something creative and clever) to show some unity, that we both agree we are all individuals, we all need to be the best version we can be and that women – when they work together – can be unstoppable.

Your Arch Enemy...'

Maria responded positively and we did both agree that our messages about health are similar and that people need to see more body diversity depicted in the media. I haven't caught up with her yet in person, but I anticipate spending some time in The States soon, and I'd like to catch up and have a chat. Who knows, we might even be able to have a healthy debate over a subject or two, I wonder if the press and TV shows would be interested in covering that?

What drove me a little bonkers about Maria Kang – the Fit Mom vs. Anti-fit Mom debate, was the thousands of women that jumped on the bandwagon that had decided the whole issue was about Woman v Woman.

Thousands of comments like these were made all over social media:

'Nothing in the world comes close to the vitriol that some women have for one another.'

'What a terrible display of the 'sisterhood' – why do women always have to pull each other down?'

'Women are such bitches.'

'She (Taryn) is just jealous of Maria Kang's body.'

'You'd never see men carry on like this, why do we women always have to get catty?'

The fact that we were two women was irrelevant. When men argue do we see headlines that infer they are going to rip each other apart wearing budgie smugglers in a mud bath? No! When two men argue, we review the debate rather than analyse any supposed gender-defined behaviour.

I didn't agree with Maria's angle of promoting health and wellbeing, but it didn't mean I hated her! Of all the things I have so far learned from the development of the Body Image Movement, one of the most important is recognising that it is fine to disagree with someone else's opinion. I see it as my role as an ambassador for positive body image to publicly encourage debate, and to question accepted stereotypical views about health and weight. I do not condone attacking others on a personal level because of their opinions. I do see my role as one of challenging the current paradigm and that does mean I will continue to disagree with certain statements promoted on social media.

Adopting this attitude of, 'I am just going to be one hundred per cent transparent, a fallible human being', changed everything for Body Image Movement. At my first speaking engagement I was a ball of nerves, but rather than disguising it with my bitch face and power suit I was just me. I took off my mask. After a few giggles, some heavy breathing and a quiver in my voice I declared to the audience, 'Thank God I have this lectern to protect me from you, I'm positively petrified right now!'

And I was. Besides speaking at Jason's funeral, I had successfully dodged and avoided most public speaking opportunities since that fateful conference presentation in Singapore, but things were different now.

Learning to open myself up and not feel compelled to be the 'expert' all the time allowed people for the first time to see the authentic me. No airs, no graces, no bullshit, no masks. So on a personal level my PR stories changed from, 'Oh we sold our second car because Mat hardly ever uses it and loves cycling to work,' to, 'Oh we sold the car because we have no money, we've poured it all into getting BIM off the ground. We're broke!'

And when the trolls had stuff to say like: 'You just want to get on *Ellen* because you want to be famous.' My response would be, 'Well, of course I want to appear on the *Ellen DeGeneres Show*, it would be a really good way to get my message out. If fame is the bi-product of this movement then maybe you're right it wouldn't be such a bad thing, because I could use my 'fame' to influence a lot of people positively!'

And to, 'You just want to make money from selling your eBook.' I say, 'Yes of course I want to make money from selling my eBook, how else am I going to pay the bills?'

So basically, with this new attitude toward my approach in developing Body Image Movement things started to flow really well and I was getting some very positive responses from my posts on social media and blogs on the website. The amount of time I was spending on the movement, however, was becoming very taxing for my family and in particular Mat. All through 2013 I was working as a photographer and using the profit I made from that to fund BIM, hence going without a second car for over twelve months, and let me tell ya, that wasn't much fun.

Every new start up business has a tale to tell but somehow mine felt harder, (insert violins and a song on the theme of 'woe is me'). The reason it felt harder was because I had just spent seven years building up a photographic business that was firing on all cylinders, and I was walking away from it to take a gamble on a 'feeling' that the world needed to hear my story.

Imagine getting that across the line with Mr Methodical Mat! 'Don't worry Mat, all will be fine, the focus must remain on helping people, I know if I do the right thing, and create BIM for the right reason some day I will be able to earn a wage.'

I worked on BIM for over a year and didn't get paid a cent and all the photography money was being spent on developing a website, creating an eBook, hosting dedicated servers, logos, flights, oh yeah and the godamned hats and t-shirts. We were positively broke, I'd already borrowed $5,000 off my Aunt to help out with the start-up costs. There was no more money. And to top it all off, the emotional strain was taking its toll on our marriage, Mat was missing his wife and I was missing my family life.

There were several times in 2012 and 2013 that I felt like walking away, but I didn't, and this was due largely to the people who supported the BIM page, a lovely bunch of strangers that I adored. I always watched award shows such as the Oscars and the Emmys when actors and filmmakers thank their fans, and I always thought it was quite disingenuous. How can they 'love' and 'thank' people they've never met? What a crock of shit I'd thought. But I get it now. I don't presume to have 'fans' per se, but the concept of feeling love and gratitude to people you've never met is very possible.

At the end of 2013 I closed my photography business so I could shift all my focus onto BIM. It was a tough and risky financial decision because up until that point all that financed the Body Image Movement were fridge magnets, an eBook and sporadic speaking opportunities. But I had to take a leap of faith so I could allow BIM to flourish as my intuition told me it would. Well-intentioned friends suggested that I leave the photography door open and use it as a fall back if BIM didn't work out, but I couldn't do that. Approaching a global movement with a safety net was not going to fly. This was all or nothing.

So I leapt, wholeheartedly and enthusiastically into the unknown. I reminded myself over and over and over that 'everything was going to be okay', that all roads had led me here, that because my intentions and purpose were so pure and genuine that the Universe would look after me. Ah the Universe! The good old Universe. Up until the time I had the epiphany I don't think that I'd ever used the word 'universe' in a sentence. Over the years when people had mentioned the Universe or their relationship with the Universe, or best still when they explained to me they 'put it out there' to the Universe, I just didn't get it. I categorised these people as either frankincense-sniffing, tree-hugging hippies or, even worse, people who had joined a cult. Now I am that 'universe' person! Not the culty video hippie version but someone who dared to believe that 'putting it out there' would reap some returns and it did... in spades.

At the beginning of 2014 I sat down and explored within myself where I wanted to take BIM, how I was going to do it and what goals I wanted to achieve. The three goals were: to begin making a documentary, to deliver a talk on TED, the influential forum for ideas worth spreading, and to meet Ellen DeGeneres. I also created a vision board that encapsulated everything that I wanted to be surrounded by, things I wanted to see and things I wanted to achieve. Amongst photos of beaches, Italy, Oprah and Ellen were words, including:

It's possible – Your time – Strong mind – The future is now – Within reach – The whole world does have to know – I have what it takes – You can be you!

I've included a photo of the board in the photo section of this book so you can check it out for yourself.

The most amazing thing started happening soon after I created this board. The things that I had put on it started to become true. Bingo, the Universe was listening! 'In print for the first time' is a reality, you're reading it now; 'Picture perfect Canada' is where I am heading to speak later in the year, and we are starting to achieve the most important two words on the board, 'Going global'.

Making the movement global was difficult, not from the perspective of reaching people all over the world, that was the easy part, the hard part was having the audacity and the temerity to actually do it.

The dark passenger in my head had been replaced with a tigress snarling, 'Who do you think you are?' After all, it's not every day you decide you're going to lead a global movement in creating change. Even when I type that I get a little twitch of discomfort! Could I do this? Could I really do this? Am I the right person for the job? Thinking about all roads that led me here, the people I'd met, the experiences I'd had, the empathy I feel, and most importantly the kind of role model I want to be for my daughter all led me to believe the answer was yes. So I said, 'fuck it'... and I went for it, the fallible female visionary with everything to lose and everything to gain.

CHAPTER NINE

The Sydney Skinny

I WAS ON THE PHONE ONE DAY to my web developer and good mate Heath Vogt. I'd met Heath through his wife at the kindergarten. One day Oliver came home with a note from another mother asking if Oliver could go to Will's house for a play date. The note more or less said that we kept missing each other and that this was the only way to make a connection. I was a little hesitant to make a friendship with someone through a note. Of course I wouldn't let Oliver go on a play date to a stranger's house without me, which meant I would have to go along too. I am not a fan of small talk and when two adults have only their children in common, all you end up talking about is boring kid talk… You could say that I completely over-thought a casual get together, and lucky for me, all my concerns were unfounded. Erica, Heath's wife, was one of the those woman that after spending some time together you start thinking, 'Mmmm how do I become her friend?' 'How do I ask my friend for her number?' (AWKWARD!) and the ultimate question, 'Could I ever meet up with my friend's friend without my friend?' SHOCK HORROR! I know you know what I mean!

Another reason I thank God I met Erica is Heath. He was invaluable in the early days of setting BIM up. When I was bleeding money, he was cutting corners and giving me good mates-rates. So I'm on the phone to Heath, and because all messages that came through my website came to him too, we both simultaneously saw a message from a Mr Nigel Marsh. We both Googled him and were so excited to have someone of his talent and influence being interested in The Body Image Movement. This is what the message said:

'Hi my name is Nigel. I am the founder of The Sydney Skinny. I would like to chat with Taryn. The objectives of The Sydney Skinny and The Body Image Movement appear to one hundred per cent aligned. Many thanks. Warm Regards. Nigel.'

Nigel Marsh is the author of three best sellers – *Fat, Forty and Fired, Overworked & Underlaid*, and *Fit, Fifty & Fired Up*. He is also the co-founder of Earth Hour (when over a billion people at the same time turn their lights off to raise awareness and funds), and the founder of the Sydney Skinny, a nude swimming event that aims to counteract negative body image issues. He also just so happens to hold the number one spot for the most watched TED talk in Australia.

Such an accomplished man! And he is contacting me. What does he want? Could he advise me about my financial woes? Does he have a proposition and what does it all mean?!

I got on the phone and tried really hard to be a super cool cat, but once I get excited, I leap from one conversational gambit to the next, often without taking a breath. Mat calls me the 'verbal machine gun'. However, Nigel coped. We spent an hour on the phone talking about The Body Image Movement, and what my plans were for the future. I explained to Nigel how difficult I was finding it to make ends meet. There was always so many unexpected bills to pay, for instance when *Good Morning America* did an interview with me my website traffic went through the roof, so I had to purchase my own dedicated server. It cost hundreds of dollars that I didn't have. It always was a deficit with Body Image Movement and while it was never about making money it was unsustainable for me to continue working for no wage. Poor Mat was at the end of his tether too. I was working every night once the kids were in bed, and there was never any time for us. I explained all this to Nigel, my new mate, someone that I'd only just been introduced to. For whatever reason I just knew that he got it.

'I am so stretched Nigel, I am under enormous amounts of pressure, I have three children and a husband, I am running two businesses – one that makes a great living that basically gets poured in to the one that doesn't make money. There is always a birthday present to buy, a dress-up day at school, the bills keep coming in, and all I want to fucking do is share my story.' Quick intake of breath and...

'I don't want to sell my soul to the devil and take a deal from the companies that are approaching me to represent them, I don't want to be a pawn in their game. I want to do this on my terms but I am getting really frustrated, I know I can help women to feel better about themselves, all I want to do is be able to pay myself a living wage...'

...and then Nigel interrupted, thank God, I was getting myself so wound up I was close to the point where there is no turning back. I'd already dropped the f bomb with a new acquaintance, who knew where I would go from there...

Nigel gave me some reassurance, 'I understand how it feels,' he said, 'I've been there too, it's tough but you just have to push through.'

And of course I knew that. The amount of times I had said to myself, 'Keep going Taz, you just have to hold on and keep going.' There were times, I told Mat and a couple of close girlfriends, that I was at the point, emotionally and physically, where most people would walk away. I could actual feel it.

Just to get a little sidetracked here (this is one of those going from one tangent things to the next, but just stay with me); in terms of people's commitment and discipline to fulfilling a goal, not all of those people that walk away are failures. In fact I don't believe that anyone is a failure. What I do know from chasing various dreams throughout my life is that sometimes when you are striving to reach a goal the reason that you walk away is because you realise you were chasing the wrong goal. That's what helped me push through to the other side of Body Image Movement, knowing that what I wanted to do was authentic and for the right reasons.

This is what Nigel and I ended up speaking about for the next half hour, being genuine and authentic. It would seem that we shared the same values when it came to body image, that we despaired of the hypocrisy in the media, and that we shared a similar disdain for people talking a big game but not delivering the results. Nigel went on to explain to me why he wanted to talk to me, and that it was at Sydney Skinny where he felt we had a combined interest.

The Sydney Skinny is the world's largest nude ocean swim, held in Cobblers Beach at the Sydney Harbour National Park. Men and women of any age can take part in the untimed, 300m or 900m swim. The aim of the swim is to celebrate unity and diversity, to combat negative body image pressure and to celebrate being alive.

Nigel filled me in on a few other details and then he said, 'It would be great to have you, given what you do with the Body Image Movement, to come along and do the swim.'

Huh? What! Me? It's one thing to be comfortable in my own skin but it's another to get starkers in front of a bunch of strangers! But Nigel went on to explain that he thought his movement and mine had a great synergy, and he would like me to not only do the swim, but also become Ambassador for Sydney Skinny. We ended the phone call with an 'I'll consider it.' The event was about nine months away so there was plenty of time to get out of it!

Nigel and I stayed in contact over the next six months or so and it was getting to crunch time, I really needed to let Nigel know what I was doing. On the way to getting dropped off to a girls lunch one Saturday afternoon, with three active kids making a bunch of noise in the back, I decided to talk to Mat about me doing the swim. I started with 'so', 'So Mat, hypothetically if I wanted to go do a nude swim in Sydney with a bunch of strangers, how would that make you feel?' The minute I asked, I was so annoyed with myself, not only for asking at a really stupid time (hello, I am going to lunch with the girls, time is limited, kids are noisy), but the way I asked it to – it was almost as if I set myself up for failure.

Mat's response; 'I don't want you swimming with a bunch of strangers naked!'

'So is the problem that I am naked or that they will see me?'

'No, I just don't want you naked around people, you're my wife.'

'Yes I know I am your wife but is it that other men will see my naked body, or that I will be surrounded by penises?'

(That was my attempt at humour, again, ten years of marriage...?)

Later that evening after a couple of glasses of champers I thought I would have another crack and see if I could persuade Mat to come around on the idea, he didn't budge. To be fair, I did see where Mat was coming from, some random dude (Nigel) rings me up and wants me to participate in a nude swim. I get it, it does sound a little tough to digest.

The Sydney Skinny was in February. It was now Christmas and I still hadn't committed one way or the other with Nigel, or got Mat's blessing. Mat was understandably feeling it was maybe a step too far. I was almost defeated. I was on a holiday with my family down at what I describe as magical Normanville (about an hour's drive from my house) and we were having a late afternoon G&T on the deck after spending the entire day in the pool. We were relaxed, the kids were happy and out of nowhere I decided to have a final crack. Just a quick FYI, Mat is a mad keen 300km a week cyclist. Here in Australia, we call them MAMILS (middle aged men in lycra!) Cycling is his great love, he is borderline obsessed, just as I am with work.

'So, Mat, you know how you adore bike riding. Well imagine how you would feel if I asked you to not ride your bike. I know this is not great timing because we are on holiday BUT I just really need you to know how much it means to me to be able to participate in the Sydney Skinny. It's not just a nude swim, it is a celebration of all that is good in this world. It is so aligned with my messaging, and I really really really want to do it. Please just have a think about how it would make you feel if I stopped you from riding, how would that feeeeeel?! Just take some time and please consider.'

That was the end of the debate, and in the New Year Mat, although not convinced, and certainly not in love with the idea, gave me the green light to do the swim. At first I was so thrilled, but then reality stepped in and that emotion turned to fear; I can't actually swim that well. Sure I could swim a couple of lengths of a pool but I've never swum 300 metres, and I only had five weeks before the race. So I rang a friend of a friend who knew of a swimming instructor and booked a session with him. His name was Marc, and he was a hilarious and very unique character.

My brief to him was that I had to swim for 300 metres straight, in five weeks without drowning in the open ocean, with thousands of other people, naked, so breaststroke was definitely off the cards.

Marc was about fifty years of age, he was gentle, encouraging and reassured me I'd be good to go in a few weeks time. I trained one on one with Marc for about three lessons and in that first week I swam every day of the week – seven days straight. It almost took me back to the bodybuilding comp days, when I had to annoyingly wash my hair endlessly.

Marc's approach to swimming was almost zen-like, in fact I referred him to a few friends as the Dalai Lama of the pool. He encouraged me to be at one with the water and not to be afraid. I remember on one occasion when he was showing me some breathing techniques (where I had to bob up and down in the water breathing normally) and he got me to close my eyes. It was the first time I felt a sense of calm in the pool. Usually when I've been around water and attempted swimming activities I would be battling for breath, and desperate gasping was a regular signature move of mine. After lessons with Marc I could swim a length of the 50m pool without feeling like I was going to die, and I felt calm and serene. It was actually really nice.

I've only ever known one speed when it comes to working out and that is hard and fast. Swimming was different, and I really enjoyed the time out of life without my phone on me. I was uncontactable, cut off for just a while, and that gave me a sense of freedom that I hadn't experienced in a long time.

Now please don't confuse how I felt swimming to how I looked swimming. You know those memes on the internet, that say with an accompanied photo, 'What I think I look like,' and then the other photo, 'What I actually look like'? I'll say no more!

February rolled around fast and I was so excited to be part of the Sydney Skinny event, I had even negotiated with Mat a four-day leave pass from life as a mother and wife so that I could spend some time helping Nigel with radio and TV interviews in Sydney.

Now Nigel is going to kill me for sharing this, but I think you'll find it funny so here I go. Nigel had arranged for me to stay in Bronte, which is just down the road from the famous Bondi Beach. Bronte is a most amazingly beautiful part of the world and visiting this suburb actually had me thinking for the first time in my life that I could live in Sydney. As a suburb, Bronte has it all, cafés, parks, a surf lifesaving club, a spectacular beach and the most amazing rock pool I've ever seen. How un-Australian of me, but I had never swum in a rock pool before, if you haven't done it, add it to your bucket list, it was truly magical. In fact Google Bronte Beach rock pool – you'll get it.

So, back to the story. Nigel had arranged for me to stay in a rental apartment in Bronte, thinking it would be nice for me to have a home away from home and in easy walking distance to the beach. When I arrived I found that the house had a well-stocked fridge, fresh food on the bench, and photographs and personal items all around the house, I found a towel and some soaps on the bed in one room and assumed that out of the two bedrooms this was the one I was meant to stay in. I unpacked my suitcase and heaved a happy sigh, this was going to be my haven for the next few days. I'd be able to kick my feet up and enjoy the solitude, maybe read a book, an entire book! Oh wow I was living the dream, four nights of peace and quiet.

I went out to grab a few staples from the supermarket. When I came back to the apartment I realised someone was in there, next thing a woman walks out of the other bedroom in just a singlet and undies and said,

'Oh hi how are you? I'm Kathy, we'll have to be quiet, Max is asleep, would you like some meatballs for lunch?'

I'm thinking, What? Who are you? Who is Max, and what are you doing here? Instead I politely replied, 'I'm good thanks, I'll just make myself a cup of herbal tea.'

Kathy: I hope you don't mind but my boyfriend is staying tonight.'

Me: 'Sure, no worries.' (HUH?!)

What is going on? I am completely and utterly confused!

Kathy and I sat down on the couch, I watched her eat meatballs and then finally plucked up the courage to admit that I was slightly confused, as I'd assumed I was staying in the apartment alone. It turns out this was Kathy's home and she rented out a room, not the entire place. Kathy was so delightful, 'Oh I feel terrible there has been this mix up, Max is a really good baby and we'll be in and out over the next few days.' As lovely as Kathy was I couldn't stay in such a small place with three other people, especially being without kids myself, I needed space. I rang Nigel and he was also taken aback. 'What a balls up, I am completely embarrassed, I'm not sure how this happened!' End of the story, I found somewhere else to stay, but there were no hard feelings and I am now friends with Kathy on Facebook, we've stayed in contact, and I am sure we met for a reason, even if that reason is only to give me a chuckle every now and again when I think of the girl in her undies and asking me if I wanted meatballs for lunch!

I woke up on the morning of the Sydney Skinny feeling slightly queasy as well as nervous. I had overindulged on Nigel's delightful wife's fish curry the night before. By now I'm sure you appreciate how much I adore food, so last night while other people around the table were thinking of their swim the next day and refusing second helpings, I was like, 'Pass it to me, this fish curry is out of this world!' And when it was dessert time, yes I indulged, yes with cream, and yes I had seconds.

I was regretting those decisions now, especially as I was getting picked up very early and there was no time for my morning Number Two. Oh dear, where and how is this going to end? I have a thing about public toilets, and nude swimming with a full tummy is disastrous!

We arrived at Cobblers Cove and I started to get butterflies. As Ambassador for the event I really had to pull my shit together, think less about myself and get out there and speak to participants. There was so much tension and anticipation in the air it was almost electric. Nigel, who is the most unassuming of men, was walking around with unshaven stubble, some crazy sandal things (it must be the Englishmen in him) and a cap. He did his thing, saying hi to everyone and anyone while most people didn't know he was the organiser and founder of the event.

It was absolutely priceless when he waved and said hello to one of the journalists from a TV station, (just like he did anyone else) and she completely snubbed him. It was pure delight for me later as we were standing at the coffee cart when she turned to me and said, 'I don't suppose you know where Nigel Marsh is?' Bingo, one of those priceless moments in life. I pointed and said, 'There he is, right there.' Her face. Oh her face!

I did a few interviews and then it was time. To get to the beach, you have to walk through the most amazing national park. It takes about five minutes, and usually it would be a place of serenity and peace, but today the sounds were of groups of people laughing and joking. It felt so good. When I got to the beach, the first thing I saw was a penis. Then I saw another, and another and another, and within minutes, a penis was just a penis and boobs were just boobs, and we were all just human beings. Nothing more: nothing less. Nothing scandalous, nothing dirty or creepy, and nothing remarkable.

I eased myself into the water and immediately felt a sense of release, pleasure and freedom. The feeling of the water on my naked skin as I glided through it was delightful. The endorphin rush of being unclothed and doing something I had never done before with a huge crowd of people was magical. This was life, and I was living it. And I wasn't alone in how I felt, I heard people squealing with joy exclaiming, 'I never want to swim with clothes on again!' and I saw others joyfully hugging as if they had just been reunited after a lifetime apart.

When I got out of the water a woman handed me a sarong and I wrapped it around me only to feel a sense of regret that it was over. I had chosen to do the 300m swim, not the 900m swim and I immediately regretted it.

I was standing there in my sarong, looking out to the ocean, and talking to a woman that I had spoken to earlier in the day about how amazing the event was, and how free and liberated we felt. Next second, out of nowhere, she shouts, 'Look over there, another woman with only one boob!' Puzzled, I turned to her and asked, 'What do you mean?' She pulled down her sarong and showed me her chest, on one side a breast, on the other side a scar. I peered in the direction she had pointed, and another woman with the same appearance was proudly walking out of the water.

I watched as two complete strangers joyfully connected with one another. No words were required, just one look of recognition, a smile and then an embrace. I was in tears, a blubbering mess. It was the purest form of human connection, kindness, courage and love and it was all unfolding before my very eyes. One of the women explained to me how big a deal it was for her to do the swim, to get naked in front of other people and to face her fear. When I asked her if she would do it again, the answer was a resounding YES!

It got me thinking that to effect a transformative change in a person's life an action is often required. (Think Anthony Robbins' method of inspiring people to break through emotional or ambitious barriers by taking part in a physical fire walk). Water is an element that has been used as a purifier in many religions. Could participation in the Sydney Skinny be the 21st century's non-religious 'psychological cleanse' that helps individuals lay their body image demons to rest? Is it possible to walk into the water with body image worries and walk out with an undeterred commitment to learn to love and respect your body more? I believe so.

Among the thousand people who were there on the day, I didn't hear one person judge anyone else. I didn't hear anyone complain or apologise about their stretch marks, cellulite or jelly belly. People were just people; there were no barriers, there was no discrimination or prejudice. People were kind to themselves and kind to each other.

I got so much more than I had bargained for when I swam the Sydney Skinny. In the course of one day my life has changed. I am a better human being and I experienced more joy than I'll ever be able to express by simply taking my clothes off and swimming in the ocean with a thousand strangers. If you ever get the opportunity to do the Sydney Skinny, don't hesitate, it will be on my calendar every year for the rest of my life. Come and say hi to me – when I've got my sarong on of course!

CHAPTER TEN

Sparkle

PARTICIPATING IN THE SYDNEY SKINNY really moved me outside my comfort zone and put me into a zone I call the 'Sparkle zone'. Now, if this was a commercial and I was standing here telling you about the Sparkle zone I would hope that you would have the self respect to change the channels. But just stay with me for a few minutes, I am not selling you anything, it's just an idea, take from it what you will.

It all started last year on my 36th birthday. I was standing in front of the mirror trimming my beard. Yes, the beard on my face. Love your body, love yourself and all that, but the hairs that are popping up all over my face, upper lip and cheeks, are somewhat annoying. I know! I must learn to 'embrace', but I nonetheless was not particularly enjoying this de-fuzz session when it occurred to me that I had lost my sparkle.

My husband had asked me earlier in the week what I would like to do for my birthday and I had responded with 'nothing'. As it turns out, I woke up and decided that I wanted to go and buy some tea towels I had seen in the local homeware store, so I rang my best friend and off we went, for a cup of coffee and some tea-towel shopping. You see, there is the evidence right there – tea towels, sparkle, not here, gone, departed. I used to be so much fun, the wild one, the party animal, the bungee jumper, the risk taker. Then I became a mum and I became the sensible one or, as officially described in my house, the 'safety officer'.

'Slow down, don't ride your bike so fast.'

'No running around the pool.'

'Don't eat too much you'll get a sore tummy.'

My days are filled with endless instructions, guidelines and requests for my children to remain safe and out of harm's way. I understand it is my duty (and one that I take very seriously) to protect and be responsible but sometimes I crave to feel like that carefree person I used to be. I miss the extreme, an element of danger, a few late nights and letting go. Going for something regardless of the consequences, streaking at a cricket match or something, anything that doesn't involve me being responsible and well-behaved!

Last year I went out dancing with the girls (one might call this clubbing but I couldn't bring myself to write it). I was having the time of my life and dancing up a storm, in my element, shaking my booty, until I realised it was 3am. I told my girlfriends I had to leave and ran out the door like Cinderella as she left the ball. I flew past some random guy who yelled to me, 'Where are you going in such a hurry?' to which I shouted back, 'I'm taking my kids to see Disney on Ice at 9am.'

I admit I had a secret puke in the toilets of Disney on Ice the next morning, but you couldn't wipe the smile off my face that day. I had got my wild fix, the old me was rejoicing and the mummy me felt back on track and ready to take on the linen cupboard for the hundredth time without too much resentment.

A few days after my not-at-all wild tea towel buying birthday treat, we were taking a week's holiday to relax with the kids and my mum and dad. It was summer and it was hot, so we decided to go to the beach. After a boogie boarding session with the boys I noticed a group of people jumping off the jetty. 'C'mon gang' I said, 'Before we head back let's go take a look at the crazy jetty jumpers.'

As we approached the jetty I noticed that all of the jumpers were either teens or very early twenties; every girl was wearing a bikini and every boy was seriously buff. I stood out like an old duck out of water, until that is, I ended up in the water. As I watched the jetty jumpers these were the thoughts going through my mind:

'Tsk, those kids are crazy, there have been at least a dozen shark sightings in this area over the past fortnight.'

'What if they landed on a sting ray and the barb stung them and killed them like poor Steve Irwin?'

'They could very easily land in an awkward position, break their spine, and end up in a wheelchair for the rest of their lives.'

'What if one of them lands on the another kid's head, they will surely break a nose or a skull?'

I'll stop there, I could in fact write an entire book just on these thoughts but I'm sure you've caught my drift.

And then this thought popped into my head, 'Sparkle, remember the sparkle. Go on, do it.' So I announced to my family that I was going to give it a crack. With a year's worth of trepidation held tightly in by my floral one-piece, I clumsily made my way up the stairs and stood at the top for what felt like an eternity. As no one now had access up or down, the traffic flow ceased and all eyes were on me.

'You guys go through, you guys come up the ladder, it's okay I'll wait. No you go first, c'mon boys go for it. Yep, you go through.'

I mean seriously, what a freaking scene I was creating, it was like I was directing traffic. Mat gave me a hurry up look. 'I can't do it', I cried down to them. 'C'mon,' my loving husband replied, 'Don't be an old woman, just do it.' And that was all it took. Spurred on by that irritating comment I went for it, jumped off the jetty, and squealed like a pig the entire way down. I emerged from the water to hear a small cheer from a group of girls (the sisterhood is still alive in the young ones; the boys just stared at me blankly) and with that one leap I had unleashed the wild beast within.

It felt so good swimming in the deep turquoise waters at the Second Valley jetty. For all I cared there were great whites and sting rays all around, I felt invincible. I'd got my sparkle fix! To appease the safety officer within I did have a really big chat to my kids about jetty jumping, the dangers of, and when it was okay and when it was not okay to do it. Cruz, my middle child has a sensory disorder, he also has an extremely high pain threshold and isn't afraid of anything. So he'll be jumping off and jumping out of anything he can, as soon as he can. It's a good thing I always give my kids a lecture on safety after I've done something particularly reckless.

One thing I did learn from this lack of sparkle, and then getting some, was the understanding that I needed to 'book in' sparkle activities. It is so easy to get caught up in the mundane everyday routine of doing what we do – making school lunches, telling kids to clean their teeth a hundred times, telling kids to open their curtains, telling kids to stop fighting, buying presents for endless birthday parties, telling kids what's for dinner, convincing kids to eat their dinner, putting a load of washing on, hanging out the washing, picking dog crap up off the back lawn, emptying the dishwasher, picking up clothes off floor, removing the crumbs from the cutlery drawer...

Sorry! I just got completely carried away, I forgot I was writing a book and thought for a moment I was in my own private therapy session. Oooo that felt good though! I know you get it, life is busy and often boringly repetitive. It is so important that we get out there and live, and enjoy ourselves, if we're lucky we are here for about eighty years, such a short amount of time. We need to embrace the sparkle!

But if engaging in sparkle feels so good then why are we not engaging with the activities that give us that rush more often? It's quite simple; humans are inherently lazy, we are creatures of habit and we don't naturally like to take risks or push ourselves into new territory. We like familiar surroundings and feeling secure and safe. And that is perfectly okay, as long as there is balance between routine and the unexpected or unusual. So I am not suggesting that we all stop working and start throwing ourselves out of aeroplanes, but that we start putting the unusual on the radar, and ensuring there is enough of the ordinary mixed up with a little of the extraordinary.

After my jetty jump I made a commitment to myself that for the next twelve months I would be proactive instead of reactive about getting my sparkle fix. I just couldn't risk getting myself so wound up that I'd get arrested at the cricket for streaking. So I pencilled in some 'sparkle' activities, starting with a stand-up paddle boarding session.

I was camping with some old friends in a place called Lorne, on the Great Ocean Road, Victoria. If you've never been, put it on your to 'places to go' list. It is the perfect blend of hippy and luxury. It has everything: surfers, cafés, fashion outlets, an awesome jetty for fishing and the most amazing coastline. My girlfriend Megan is a regular stand-up paddle boarder and she had promised to take me out for my first time. We left the kids at the campsite with the dads and cruised off in her dual cab, with surf board on top – I was all smiles and getting a sense of the sparkle before we'd even got to the beach.

When we'd got into our wetsuits (we were so *Point Break*), Megan said she'd go out first and show me some techniques. The water was choppy but once she got past the break, she stood up and she was paddling, she made it look so relaxing and effortless. By the time she made it back to shore half an hour later, the seas had got even rougher we agreed that it wasn't a good idea for a first timer to challenge the waves. Disappointed we started walking back to the car when I noticed a little inlet of water. 'Hey Megs, check out that water over there.' It was perfectly calm and there were a few people fishing from the bridge above, the water was very still. We headed over and agreed that this was the perfect place to learn to paddle board. I paddled around on my knees for about half an hour, I must have been a real sight for the fishermen. I passed one and I said to him, 'I really want to stand up but I think I might fall in!' He replied 'Yeah, you don't want to fall into this water!' which I thought was odd, but I didn't think much of it and continued paddling around the water balanced safely on my knees. About ten minutes later I went from knees to feet and I was stand up paddling! I let out a loud 'WOO HOO' much to the dismay of all the people fishing who were looking at me strangely. Oh well, that's their problem, I thought, I'm having a date with sparkle and no one can stop me! Eventually I called it quits, the water was so black and with the sun going down, it was time to call it a day.

Megan and I hugged on the bank of the river, my feet sinking into the dirty combination of green grass and mud. She was delighted that I felt so good. We picked up the board and the paddle and started making our way back to the car. You'll never guess what we saw on the way. Not one, two, or three, not even four but FIVE warning signs to keep out of the HIGHLY CONTAMINATED WATER. Oh my God! I thought, that's why the fishermen were all looking at me weirdly as I cheerily waved to them while wobbling on my board. Thank goodness I didn't fall in.

I immediately got back to the campsite and took a shower. I have a severe phobia of gastro problems and the thought of my body coming into contact with contaminated water made me feel quite uneasy!

A quick side story for you, my fear of gastro bugs stems from a traumatic experience when I was 37 weeks pregnant with Mikaela. I had to be taken to the hospital because I had been vomiting for hours and had become quite dehydrated. When I arrived at the hospital (which is on a main road and it was peak hour) I climbed out the car and fell to my knees and starting vomiting on the footpath. To top it off a little bit from the other end came out too. You could imagine I was a sight for sore eyes for people driving to work, a heavily pregnant women on all fours, vomiting on the footpath. Mat had run into the hospital to get some help and came back with a wheelchair, I snapped at him, 'I don't want that, I'll walk, I've just shit my pants I can't sit down.' A drip for twenty-four hours and I was back on track, with another poo story to tell for drunken evenings around the campfire!

Back at the Lorne campsite, I prayed to the gastro gods that no osmosis occurred with the water and my body, Mat just laughed 'You're not a plant Taryn!' But nothing could wipe the smile off my face, I had got my fix of sparkle and it felt good!

This year I have lots of other sparkle activities lined up, including a couple of trips to the nudist beach for a swim, horse riding, a triathlon (it's very small but a triathlon nonetheless!) abseiling and meditating in Bali. I've already survived downhill mountain biking (only just!), coaching the under eight's soccer team and going wakeboarding for the first time, it's been a good start to the year. I am so excited for what the future holds. And now I challenge you. Go out and find your sparkle. Try something new this year that pushes your boundaries.

CHAPTER ELEVEN

The before and after photos

AT THE TIME OF WRITING this chapter it is the first day of my period. Day One is never pleasant, there's some leftover PMT and irritability from the week before, I have cramps, and my eyes are a little fuzzy. What a fab day to be writing about a bunch of fucking arseholes, oops, I mean what a day to be writing about an interesting group of people with different opinions.

The first time I truly experienced the wrath of the internet trolls was when I posted my non-traditional 'before and after' photos. On that particular day, I had been to watch and support some new friends that I had met on my brief bodybuilding journey, who were competing in their first competition. Talking afterwards the main topic of conversation was how they were going to love their bodies now, after their peak had been achieved, and the only way was down? What they were saying was basically true, if you are only judging the physical form of the body, and if your values dictate that minimum fat is the only currency of the perfect body. I tried to explain to them in ten minutes how I felt about my body and what I had had to do to get to that place, hugged them, wished them well and headed home.

Later that evening, when I was thinking about the girls wondering how they'd feel about their less than perfect bodies, an idea popped into my head. I would post a different kind of before and after weight loss photograph, the before shot would be me onstage in the fitness competition, and the after would be a photo that had been taken by my girlfriend Kate Ellis just a few months previously.

Kate was a photographer and I had asked her to take some photos of me to use for biographies and that sort of thing. I also had it in my head that I would write a book one day called, 'Hotdogs and nipples the size of dinner plates', so to this photoshoot I brought along dinner plates and... wait for it, Frankfurter sausages. For some very strange and reason I thought it would be funny to put the sausage between the two folds of my stomach, making it look like a hotdog. Oh how wrong I was!! The photos were a complete disaster, I think we took about three and swiftly decided that the 'hotdog' photos were all sorts of wrong, on every level! I've bravely for the first time (ever) shared one of those photos in the photo section of the book – purely there for YOU to have a giggle.

When it comes to the creative impulse, sometimes the ideas in your head and their realisation can be two very different things. At least I gave my darling friend Kate a very good laugh that day, and best of all we got the 'after' photo, unknowingly at the time. I had had these photos sitting on my hard drive for months and I hadn't done anything with them. So that night, when the idea for the before and after photos came into my head, I immediately knew the perfect 'nudey' photo to use.

So around 9.30pm on a Sunday night, I posted the photographs with this text:

'Here are my non-traditional 'before' and 'after' photos. Traditionally when we see a 'before' photo, the person is represented as sad, overweight and quite miserable (sometimes even holding a newspaper). Miraculously in the 'after' photo once they have shed a few pounds they are blissfully happy, confident and self-assured. Have we become conditioned to thinking that we should only love our body when it's in 'perfect condition'?

I just wanted to share with you that I loved my body on that stage, prancing around in a bikini as much as I loved my body when I was sitting butt naked in my girlfriend's studio. Our bodies will go through many changes in our lives. Our bodies change through ageing, pregnancy, illness, weight loss, weight gain the list goes on. One thing we must learn to do is love our bodies before, during and after...

Be loyal to your body, love your body, it's the only one you've got.'

And within seconds I just knew that the post struck a chord because the likes went through the roof. By the time I went to bed there was over one thousand likes. When I woke up the enormity of the photos really hit home, there were thousands of likes and hundreds of comments and shares, but among the positive responses were a few really vitriolic negative comments that really shocked me. It was my first experience of dealing with nasty comments.

She's not gross, but if looking average is your goal than good for you.

Sucks to be your husband. Bloke thought he was doing alright for himself than you became a fat overweight pig.

Big is ugly. You are big now, therefore you are ugly now!

Before picture: arteries normal. After picture: arteries blocked ... No excuse for being fat! Beauty is on the inside... Doesn't mean you have to neglect your body.

Gross, fat, overweight, why do women need to let themselves go?

What a pig, why would you post this photo of yourself? You should be embarrassed by it.

This after picture of this woman is definitely NOT healthy! I can see why larger women would think so though. She is obviously overweight, and whoever thinks she looks healthy in her after pic needs to do a little more research and book reading, and a little less sittin' on the couch and snacking. You should really cover up your body, it is not nice to look at.

Admittedly these negative comments were few, only about five per cent compared to ninety-five per cent of positives, but being under fire took me right back to my high school days, being bullied and unfairly harassed. All I wanted to do was hit back, in fact I was positively BUSTING to reply to the trolls. For a number of reason

I didn't. Firstly, the trolls were actually helping me to get more eyeballs on BIM. Secondly, the trolls would love nothing more than for me to engage with them because getting a response means they win. Thirdly, I knew I had a long road ahead with Body Image Movement, it wouldn't have been proper or responsible of me to stoop to their level and get scrappy.

I needed to show restraint and maturity – bah that was hard. Ever since school I had made a conscious decision to stand up for myself, I wouldn't let anyone run all over me. So to sit back and 'take it' was difficult, my natural instincts wanted to fight back, but I just couldn't. I never responded and thank goodness I didn't, but sometimes I allow myself to fantasise about what I would have said to some of these gits. This is how I would have loved to respond:

'YOU ARE FAT AND LAZY'

Listen up bozo, how dare you judge me. I am fit, healthy, I run, I climb up mountains, I can even don lycra and keep up with the peloton, there ain't nothing lazy about me, you fucking asshole.

'YOU ARE A BAD ROLE MODEL TO YOUR CHILDREN'

How dare you comment about what sort of parent I am based on one photo, you don't know what sort of parent I am, you don't know the first thing about me – you fucking asshole.

'YOU ARE PROMOTING OBESITY'

Listen up dickhead, I'm promoting a positive body image, have you not noticed that bodies come in all shapes and sizes? Oh, yeah, you're a fucking asshole too.

I imagine it would be quite fun to be able to say whatever I pleased when I pleased, I am sure it would feel like Julia Robert's character Vivienne in the movie *Pretty Woman*, when she goes back into the clothes shop that wouldn't serve her and says, 'Big mistake. Big. Huge.' I am sure retribution and revenge feels sweet but there is just no room for that in my public life with Body Image Movement.

The before and after photos received a lot of attention in the media – in Australia and right across the world. A few days after I posted them I received a phone call from Channel 9's live *The Today Show* wanting to interview me about the Body Image Movement and the before and after photo. 'Yes, yes, yes!' I enthusiastically squealed, so eager, so incredibly eager! I'd never been on TV before and I was most excited about being given the opportunity to share my message with millions of women across the country.

When I found out about the TV interview I was camping with my family in Robe, a delightful seaside town about four hours from Adelaide. On the way home we decided to take the kids to see the Naracoorte caves, South Australia's only World Heritage site and as far as caves go, simply stunning. As with any tourist spot, the caves had a souvenir shop and a café where I bought a chicken pie. The woman at the counter warned me it was hot, but disregarding her completely I took a big reckless bite of the pie, and... 'Yeaaoooooowwwww FAR OUT!'

The pie burnt my chin and lips, severely. I couldn't stop going on and on, 'Mat this is bad, this is really bad.' Mat responded with his standard sarcastic, 'Do you want me to ring the ambulance?'

'No Mat, this pie has burned me, I am going on TV in three days!'

That pesky chicken pie gave me little burns on my face that looked like cold sores but they were the least of my worries. I was beyond nervous about being interviewed and spent days on the toilet with nervous Number Ones and Twos. When I arrived in Sydney I was picked up at the airport by a man with my name on a board, woo fancy! And he carried my bags and drove me in a pimped out Audi to my hotel. That night I stayed up until after midnight practising what I would say in front of the mirror.

The next morning was 2 May, the anniversary of the day my brother had passed away ten years before, in Sydney, so I felt emotional arriving in the same city to say the very least. But I had to park any of those thoughts because I had a job to do, I had to stay off the toilet long enough to string a few sentences together and make myself sound like a normal and together human being – not an easy gig when you're as nervous as I was!

My friend and colleague at Body Image Movement, Dr. Emma Johnston's last words to me before I got on the plane for the interview was, 'Taz, don't fuck this up, no one will want to work with you if you don't get this right!' Wow, Emma, cheers! We've been friends since our firstborns arrived, so we knew each other really well and she could get away with speaking so bluntly. She was right though, I did have to do a good job.

Speaking of doing a good job – wow those makeup girls really know how to cover up chicken pie burns don't they? What a stellar job they did. With makeup applied and locks brushed it was time to go on set and tell my story.

I was hiding behind some big black curtains pacing up and down trying to get a handle on my nerves, when the curtains were flung back by Ben Fordham, a presenter on the show. 'What are you doing behind here?'

'Oh I just feel really nervous and I am trying to pull it together,' I responded.

'Well come out of there for starters, listen you are going to be positively fine. The best thing you can do is smile and give lots of energy.' I agreed and then he said, 'Anyway, it doesn't really matter what you say, they'll just remember you for being the girl in the cool red and orange glasses.' And he laughed, gave me a high five and walked away. It was a random moment, but one that I am grateful for having. If Ben hadn't found me behind the curtain I might have missed my call on set.

It was really strange being on the set of a TV show that I've watched for years. There were people everywhere, the lights were bright and there was a flurry of activity going on all around. Georgie Gardener was interviewing me, I shook her hand and sat down opposite her. Her smile was warm and friendly. I was desperately trying to get my breathing to slow down, but all I could manage was fast and shallow. Oh well, I thought, at least I'm breathing!

In front of us was a teleprompter with my before and after photos, while looking at me, but speaking to her producer in her earpiece, Georgie said,'The photos are back to front.'

'No no Georgie, they're not.' I butt in on her conversation to the invisible producer, 'That's the whole point, they are my non-traditional before and after photos. In an attempt to get women to love their bodies I flipped the usual photos around...'

Next minute a man starts yelling a countdown, 10, 9, 8...

I feel completely and utterly panicked and turn to Georgie and say, 'This is my first time on TV, Georgie, I'm freaking out, I'm so nervous!'

6, 5, 4...

Then Carl, the presenter of the show, out of nowhere, starts yelling, 'C'mon Taryn let's feeeeeeel your energy!' His fist pumping like a crazy man! I start to chuckle, I see Ben who gives me a thumbs up, and then I hear...

2, 1...

And we were on! Live!

I did stumble on the first few words, but after about thirty seconds I was feeling more at ease, in fact crazily enough I was enjoying myself! And as the interview came to a close I thought to myself, 'Dammit that's gone too quick, I have so much more to say!'

As we were walking off the set I turned to Georgie and said, 'Georgie you're a mum, any chance you could give me a mummy hug?' And she did! So there we were, Georgie and I hugging it out in the middle of *The Today Show* set. Hilarious. Poor Georgie probably thought I was a little odd, but she was delightful, giving me some strong words of encouragement and wishing me the very best for The Body Image Movement.

The interview was successful, thank goodness, because TV appearances were something that I would have to get used to doing on a regular basis, apparently my story was newsworthy. It felt strange and unusual to have so much attention focused on me, and it would take some getting used to.

CHAPTER TWELVE

You are promoting obesity!

LAST YEAR I APPEARED ON *SUNRISE,* another live morning television program. The segment was on body image and I was sharing my story and the message of celebrating diversity and body confidence. As with all of my television interviews I was really nervous leading up to the four-minute interview but the second it was over I wanted more!

Sunrise showcased a bunch of my photos including the before and after photos, and the photo where I am covering my boobs with the dinner plates.

I was staying in Sydney for the evening so I decided to take myself out to the pub for dinner. Because I travel for work a lot, dining alone is something that I'm used to doing and doesn't faze me in the slightest, apart from one time in Christchurch when I decided to try oysters for the first time. I am not exactly sure what I was thinking but I ordered a dozen oysters, raw, as an appetiser. Yes, you read correctly, a dozen, and yes, raw and yes it was my first time. What was I thinking? I put the first one in my mouth and dry retched so loud that other diners looked across at me. It was the one time I really pined for someone to be sitting opposite me that could've laughed off the moment with me, or at least eaten a few of my oysters! Not willing to admit defeat or waste food, or send back perfectly good oysters, with great difficulty I made my way through five of them. Suffice it to say that the next morning I was vomiting out oysters in the toilets. Very unpleasant!

So there I was, solo, in Sydney, at the pub eating a nice safe burger and reading through the Facebook comments on the *Sunrise* page, and this is what some people had to say about the story and my photos:

'How attractive, fat and stretch marks, cover that up, I just ate.'

'A lot of fat women use having given birth to children as an excuse... that's the reality.'

'Sorry, I don't like it. I don't think it's attractive or appropriate.'

'There is clearly a fat epidemic that there never used to be. It's from lack of exercise except when lifting hand to mouth. Stop being PC and just say it how it is... no excuses.'

'Sorry but you're overweight you don't have curves. That's just excess fat hanging of your body.'

'Embracing Big Macs more like it.'

Could you imagine eating a burger and reading those comments? If it hadn't been so good and if I hadn't been enjoying it so much, I might have spat it out!

I understand that trolls lurk around social media waiting for an opportunity to put their nasty pants on and take someone down. I've experienced them before but on this particular occasion they got on my goat. There was a reoccurring comment that kept cropping up, it wasn't the standard, 'You're gross, fat, disgusting, ugly, a pig,' it was much worse. It was, 'You are promoting obesity.'

How the fecking heck am I promoting obesity? I am promoting body love and body acceptance for all people, small, big, short, wide, tall, soft, curvy and thin – it doesn't matter what your body shape is, everyone has a right to a positive body image.

The worst thing about the promoting obesity comments was that they didn't come from trolls, the people making these comments appeared to be average people sharing their opinions. If the comment 'you are promoting obesity' had only occurred a handful of times I'd probably not be too concerned but it was coming up over and over again. If I'm completely honest years ago I might've looked at someone who was grossly overweight and judged them as being unhealthy. This is what I was told to be true growing up, this is what I saw in the media, on billboards, and this is what doctors told us. Now I know this NOT to be true. I now know that you cannot necessarily judge anyone's health by their appearance.

Take my brother, for example. If you had met Jason on the street, most people would've described his appearance as being healthy, athletic and strong. The reality was that he was far from healthy. His young body was suffering and he was injecting himself with heroin daily. If I stood Jason side-by-side with an 'overweight' person and asked one hundred people to take a guess who out of the two was healthier, I bet Jason would've had the most votes hands down.

That's because as a society, we judge, we categorise, we stereotype. Bigger people are often labelled as lazy, undisciplined and passive, while thinner people are labelled as superficial, confident and vain. We need to stop the instant judging and we should stop commenting on how people look.

Just a few weeks ago I was talking to a woman who told me that she had always been thin, she was thin as a child and she was thin now as an adult. Growing up girlfriends would often call her a skinny bitch, thinking they were being complimentary. 'It hurt me deeply,' she said, 'And since then I've had a complex about being too thin. Now imagine if I called them a fat bitch, I wonder how they would feel?'

I watched her tell me this story with sad eyes, and with her voice quivering ever so slightly, but enough for me to notice. Her body was judged and she took those judgements with her into adulthood, would those feelings of not being good enough ever leave her? I doubt it.

As a society we need to adopt a zero tolerance policy on body shaming of any sort and we must consider that health is not just physical health but emotional and spiritual too. Spiritual health for me is having a sense of wholeness and a connection with others, and emotional health means feeling in control of my thoughts, behaviour and feelings. But because we can't always see spiritual or emotional health it doesn't seem to rate as high as physical health.

I remember when my body was transforming during the body competition training, and everyone around me praised me for being so amazing and inspirational. That's because they just judged me for what I looked like. When does weight loss equal inspirational? I didn't get it. If my emotional and spiritual health was on 'show' then they might have reconsidered their high evaluation of inspiration.

During training for the competition I felt more alone than I'd ever felt, I was self-obsessed and certainly not connected with the world, in fact I think it's fair to say that I lived in my own world for those fifteen weeks. To give you an understanding of how disconnected I was from normal thoughts during my training, I will share a story with you – even though I'm embarrassed to share it.

It was the Thursday night before the competition and I was driving in my car, turning right at an intersection. The traffic lights went orange so I started to creep forward and then out of nowhere a car sped up and ran a red light. I had to slam on my brakes hard, and he swerved aggressively only to miss my car by centimetres. With the speed he was going, and the angle of my car, if he had connected I would most certainly have ended up in hospital, no question.

The first thought I had was, 'Oh my God I wouldn't have been able to compete.'

Now just digest that for a second. I am a wife, and a mother of three young children, wouldn't you assume that my first thoughts would be of my safety for the sake of my family? Nope. My first thought was being able to be in a fitness competition. I was out of balance, physically I might've appeared to look healthy but scratching at the surface would reveal a person with a compromised spiritual and emotional health.

Because I spend my life talking to people I have heard many stories from many women who have felt that their health has been unfairly judged by their appearance. Last year I was talking to a friend who is raising two sons on her own. We were discussing health and she said to me, 'Taryn, right now I cannot focus on anything other than my emotional health. Yes I am overweight, yes I could be fitter, but right now I am JUST managing to keep my mental shit together.'

And then there are the women that have been sexually abused as children and have used food to cope emotionally with their lives. I've heard some of their stories and it's nearly killed me, the horror that some of these people have lived through, not only as a child but for a lifetime. Could you imagine surviving child abuse and then spending the next twenty years being ridiculed and being called fat, lazy and obese?

These women might be considered 'overweight' but who are we to judge them and their choices. The women I've spent time with often have a desire to be more physically healthy, they want to weigh less, but they are so focused on surviving their day from an emotional health perspective that the idea of heading to the gym and eating a salad is just not on their radar.

It's because of these women that on some occasions, when the trolls come out to comment, I just want to fight them. Not for me, call me names, whatever, but these comments negatively impact other women, the amount of times I've heard, 'Wow, if they think you're fat and gross imagine what they would think of me?'

Wouldn't it be great to take fat back to being a noun rather than an adjective. We have fat, we are not fat, just like we have fingernails but we are certainly not fingernails! But fat and fat people are treated like terrifying news headlines. OBESITY! EPIDEMIC! NEW HEALTH WARNINGS! Fat is bad. If you are fat you are lazy and fat will kill you – well, not necessarily. Would you be surprised if I told you that studies have shown that fat people are not dying from being fat, in fact on average 'overweight' people live longer than 'normal' weight people? It's almost as good as the other myth – if you lose weight you will live longer. Really? Show me the research paper on that one, you won't find it because there isn't one. All that society's increasingly panic-stricken attitude towards 'the obesity epidemic' has done is heighten levels of anxiety and depression and distorted our attitude toward body diversity.

Imagine if you lined up one hundred six-month old babies in a row, would they all look the same? No! Some would be small, others tall, some wider, some shorter, some with hair, some without, there would be no two babies that looked the same, that's because we are all uniquely different packages. We all come in different shapes and sizes, so why is it when we grow up we are put under pressure to conform to one body shape?

Personally, I think it is greed and profit that drives this conformity. Imagine a world where people embraced their bodies for what their bodies looked like, that is my dream world! Imagine a world without diets? I always encourage people to steer clear of any word in which the first three letters spell 'die'. I like to consider it a sign.

I have been on every diet you can possibly imagine, I'm talking low carbohydrate diets, high protein diets, food combining diets, fruit only diets, calorie restricted diets; if a diet exists, I have been on it. And if you measure a diet's success by a lack of kilos put on, then I have failed every diet! That's because those little fuckers don't work. Let me repeat that DIETS DON'T WORK! A recent study showed that a staggering ninety-five per cent of dieters who lost weight put the weight back on and even more alarming, two thirds of those people ended up heavier than they were before. We've got more diets than we've ever had and a greater rate of obesity, FIGHTING fat hasn't made the fat disappear!

It's time to raise the white flag because we've officially lost the war on obesity. We need to look at ourselves and our health from another perspective. What the world doesn't need is another slim-down shake or 'diet expert', what the world needs is a self-love overhaul. Oh dammit that will never work (said in my most sarcastic voice) there's no money in that! The power of change lies within each of us, it's just a shame that so many womens' self worth is determined by a number on a scale.

And just while I'm in rant mode, can I please urge you if you have a set of scales to ditch them? Your health cannot be determined by a number. And don't you think it's a little odd allowing a number to dictate your mood for the rest of the morning or the day?

Back in the day when I thought scales were my best mate, I would weigh myself every day, naked, after my morning wee and before breakfast. Weighing myself was part of my morning routine, just like having a shower or brushing my teeth, I never forgot to do it. From the moment I stepped onto the scales I was judging myself, was I fat or thin, good or bad, had I succeeded or failed. How crazy was that? Allowing a few numbers on a square shaped object to be so influential on my level of self-worth and my mood for the day.

Ditching my scales was incredibly liberating. Having spent so much time at Weight Watchers over the years and weighing myself daily, I was amazed at the sense of freedom that throwing away one small object could do for me. When I encourage women to get rid of their scales I get looked at like I am speaking a foreign language, how could I endorse such a radical thing?!

So now that we've established that scales are bad, and diets don't work, how are we going to fight back against the multibillion dollar food and diet industries that would like us to believe what they say, and who line their pockets with our money? It's time to get educated and take a collective stand to say, 'enough is enough'.

There's a movement I strongly support that I hope will help to balance the negative mainstream attitudes to size and weight, called Health At Every Size. This is a scientifically valid program based on extensive research that shows that size does not determine health status. In her book of the same name, Dr. Linda Bacon discusses at length the detrimental and harmful effects of dieting and weight loss. She also discusses the politics of the weight loss and diet industry, saying that research needs to be understood in the context of how it was funded. Research that indicates there is an 'obesity epidemic' has been funded by pharmaceutical companies that make a great deal of money from weight loss medications and other treatments. In fact, the research that led to the conclusion that obesity is the number one cause of preventable death was discovered to be misleading in its interpretations.

I feel that the statement that obesity is killing us must be seen as false when we recognise that as a society we are become somewhat fatter, but at the same time our life expectancy has increased dramatically, and chronic diseases appear later in life than before. Therefore the incremental increases in weight have not had a detrimental effect on our overall health.

As discussed by Dr. Bacon, we hear that being overweight or obese puts our health at significant risk, however when we examine studies that control for factors such as fitness, activity levels, weight cycling and socioeconomic status, there is no increased risk of disease in people who are overweight or obese. Another fabrication that we are fed as a society is that anyone who is determined enough can lose weight and keep it off. The fact is that, for various reasons, ninety-five per cent of people who lose weight regain some or all of that weight, which often leads to weight cycling that can significantly compromise health.

The most important message in terms of overweight and obesity is that health indicators can be improved through behaviour change, irrespective of our size. As Emma Johnston, the BIM Clinical Psychologist says, we need to be able to love our body as it is now, to enable us to nurture it through health and wellness activities. Hating our body does not motivate us to change behaviours. Loving our body and appreciating it for what it can do now, in recognition of the journey our body has been on, does motivate change.

So am I promoting obesity through the vehicle of the Body Image Movement? Of course not. I am promoting self respect, nurturing true appreciation for our bodies, and embracing body diversity.

CHAPTER THIRTEEN

The newsagency

NOT LONG AFTER THE FITNESS COMPETITION I was browsing the magazine rack at my local newsagency when I overheard a conversation between three girls behind the counter. I was looking for a cosmetic surgery magazine for research purposes and ironically they were discussing their impending cosmetic surgery. I found the magazine I was after but had to pretend to be looking for something else, as their conversation was getting more and more interesting. It was the one and only occasion I was actually grateful for the lack of service in a retail situation.

Two of them were talking about the surgery they had scheduled in Thailand in a few months time and the other was considering the options of getting preventative Botox.

I had been lurking around the magazines for ten minutes, it was getting awkwardly long, I felt compelled to fess up and talk to the girls. I walked to the counter and said, ' Hi girls, sorry, but I've been eavesdropping on your entire conversation about cosmetic surgery, I am completely intrigued as to why three young girls would want to get surgery?'

Thank goodness they were nice and giggly girls as opposed to the 'mind your own beeping business' kind! The one thinking of having Botox was seventeen years old, the others were nineteen and twenty-one. They were extremely open to my questions and I soon found out that the older girls were going to Thailand to get boob jobs because it was cheap and basically because 'they could'. They were so nonchalant about the surgery because so many of their friends had done it, and after all, it really wasn't a big deal. 'But what is wrong with your body as it is now?' I asked one of the girls.

She responded, 'I'm flat chested and the boys don't like a girl with no boobs.' I just wanted to rescue her right then and there and give her a big lecture about self worth, the risks of surgery and the fact that any boy that judged her for her breast size was not worth it. But this wasn't the time for one of my rants. We were standing in their place of work, after all.

I asked the seventeen-year-old about her plans to get preventative Botox, and she replied, 'All the mums do Botox and I've read that if you do it early you won't get any wrinkles.'

'What's wrong with wrinkles?' I asked.

'They make you look old!'

'And what is wrong with looking old?'

It reminded me of the countless times I was asked when working as a photographer, 'Can you please Photoshop my wrinkles.' I can honestly say that in nearly all photoshoots that involved a woman I was asked to 'enhance' her photos in some way. Sometimes it was in jest, but the subject of Photoshopping nearly always got a mention. It was only after I closed my photography business that I was able to reflect on each of the jobs I did with families, and the language that mothers so often used. It was really sad to hear mother after mother after mother say, 'Oh I don't want to be in the photos,' or 'Let's just have a couple of me and the rest of the kids,' and this old chestnut, 'I don't like having my photo taken.' Why, why, why, you beautiful creature, giver of life, you divine goddess – wouldn't you want to have your photo taken?

It made me think, is it any wonder that the girls in the newsagency wanted to change themselves when so many female role models around them, probably including their own mothers, hated the way they looked?

I thank God that I grew up in a more accepting era. My childhood was untarnished by unrealistic body ideals, all I wanted to do was roller-skate with my friends and ride my bike to the shops. But for girls these days the pressures to conform to the notion of a beauty ideal is driving them to surgery, eating disorders, body dysmorphic disorders and depression. When a girl wants to look like the girl in the magazine, but the photograph isn't an honest representation of the model, then we have a big problem on our hands.

Last week I was attacked by the Photoshop brush, without my consent. My photo was taken for a newspaper and at the time the photo was taken I had gigantic cold sore. I posed, I smiled and I didn't give my herpes lip a single thought. The next day I opened up the newspaper and there I was, full colour, half page – flawless. Without a cold sore is what I mean – I just laughed at the irony of my image getting digitally enhanced.

Tina Fey (the American comedian) once wrote, 'Photoshop itself is not evil. Just like Italian salad dressing is not inherently evil, until you rub it all over a desperate young actress and stick her on the cover of Maxim, pretending to pull her panties down. Give it up. Retouching is here to stay. Technology doesn't move backward. No society has ever de-industrialized.'

I agree that Photoshop is not evil when used in a responsible manner, but when it's used to create thigh gaps and slice off natural hip width from a woman, that's when I have a problem.

At the newsagency that day there was something else that caught my attention. When I was spending my time listening to the girls' conversation but pretending to look through magazines, I noticed an alarming difference between the covers of the boys' magazines and the cover of the girls' magazines. The words on the boys' mags said things like: 'High adventure awaits', 'Take the plunge', 'Action plus'.

While the girls' covers said: 'Get a hot mane makeover', 'Look flawless', 'One-minute makeovers'.

Notice something a little alarming? Boys are encouraged to get out and live and be adventurous while girls are encouraged to focus on their looks. For many young girls, the importance of looking good fast becomes the benchmark measure for success, and when girls internalise this concept and embrace it to be true, they spend their lives obsessing over their looks and spending abhorrent amounts of money on their external beauty.

When I grew up, there was no social media, no selfies, no Photoshop, I played cricket in the middle of the street and when a car was coming we'd all yell 'caaaaaarrrr' and move our stumps to the curb before resuming. I am not saying that we didn't have pressure to look or be a certain way but it wasn't all consuming like it is for the young girls of this generation. As a kid I wasn't sitting around waiting for 'likes' on a posted photo on Instagram, I was out at the gorge looking for frogs, and rather than heading to the beauty salon at the age of fourteen I was going on adventures with my friends on our bikes. I'm not saying I had the perfect childhood or I was the perfect child, sheesh by no means, I spent plenty of time smoking behind the deli and sneaking in a drink at the school social, but I wasn't hung up on what I looked liked, or how I was being perceived, or whether or not I was an object of desire. I feel a sense of sadness for girls growing up now in the state that the world is currently in, they don't have the sense of freedom and lack of care that we seemed to enjoy as kids.

Since that day in the newsagency, I've spent a lot of time with young girls discussing their world, and I'm not only saddened by the stories I've listened to, I am ENRAGED by the pressures they feel they are under to conform and 'be normal'. I want to share with you some stories about the vagina. The vagina has three primary functions, one is sexual intercourse, one is as the passageway for menstrual blood, the other is for childbirth. My vagina has served me very well, it has been on the receiving end of some good times over the past twenty years and has birthed three of my children. I am proud of my vagina, just like a runner is proud of their legs for running a race or a heart transplant patient is proud of their beating heart after surgery.

The problem for young girls today is that they are not proud of their vaginas, in fact they are doing all they can to change them and make them look better or even sparklier. Yes, I am referring to vajazzling; put down the studded diamonds – you are sparkly enough!

Pubic hair is a marketers dream. I know of a mum whose young teenage girls insisted she get a 'Brazilian' wax (removal of all hair) because they wanted her to 'fit in' with other girls' mums. Turning what is a very normal part of the human body into something dirty and 'unwanted' is driving girls to dislike their natural body. I also wonder if part of the problem is the way in which children can so easily access pornographic material now. Pornography is so gynaecological in this day and age, with nothing left to the imagination. This perhaps leads to a problem of a lack of vaginal diversity in pornographic material, not to mention the expectations that both boys and girls may develop about sex.

But why stop there? It's not enough telling girls that their pubic hair is gross, now they are also being told that sweating is embarrassing. There is ad on TV in Australia that makes my blood boil every time I see it. It's an ad for a sports liner and it depicts three women working out, one is boxing, the other is in an aerobics class and the last one is on the beach running. In all three examples, the girl is smashing out her workout, looking fierce and in the zone, UNTIL she looks down and notices that she has a sweat patch in her pubic area. Each girl is mortified, the two girls in the gym scenario run out of the gym and the girl at the beach runs straight into the water. 'OH MY GOODNESS, THE HORROR OF SWEATING DOWN ... THERE!' Seriously, what a crock of 'let-me make-you-feel-insecure-so-you-will-buy-my-product' shit. When we work out, we sweat, it is what our body is designed to do, there is nothing wrong with sweat on your face, or under your arms, or on your legs, or in your pubic area.

For as long as I can remember, the vagina has been a dirty word. On my speaking circuit I always try to tweak my presentation so that I can sneak in a few words about the vagina! I want to dispel the myths, and just as we celebrate our heart for pumping blood, and our lungs for breathing air, I would love women and young girls to celebrating their vagina – for reproducing, for pleasuring and for allowing us to give childbirth. I also like to throw in randomly (when the crowd is right!) that no woman or girl should wear a sports liner, not until we see BALL liners on the market.

But that will never probably happen right? Because there are a different set of rules for girls and boys. I appreciate that boys have a set of their own pressures, including the desire to be tough and strong, and steroid use in young men is becoming an increasing concern, but it's our girls that I worry about the most. The result of women and young girls being perceived as nothing more than sexual objects is giving rise to a culture of rape and abuse.

If you want to see for yourself what is going on, just go online and take a look at the violence that is perpetrated against women in mainstream video games. It makes me sick to my stomach. In 2008 a version of the hugely popular video game *Grand Theft Auto* was released in which players had the option to increase their points by sexually assaulting prostitutes. That version of the game was withdrawn in Australia, and a new censored version was later released, but this kind of attitude is worryingly commonplace.

There are many less graphic examples of sexualising young girls and objectifying women in the media, you only need to flick through a magazine or look at a billboard to find them. There's a seminar I have developed called Developing Daughters, Supporting Sons with my colleague Clinical Psychologist Emma Johnston, which I deliver to groups of parents to encourage them to help foster a positive body image in their children. We often hear gasps of horror when we show the audience images that we find every day in magazines. For example an image that depicts two woman snorting up a dress that is made to look like cocaine (selling clothes), or an ad where a woman looks like she is going to be gang raped by a group of six men (again selling clothes) or the several images I have of young women sucking provocatively on a lollipop, selling anything from a handbag to perfume.

The thing is, when I ask the question whether this sort of advertising is acceptable I always get a resounding NO as a response. We don't want it. We don't like it! So why does our disdain towards the sexualisation and objectification of women in advertising fall on deaf ears? Why doesn't someone do something about it?

If we left it up to the advertisers and the companies selling this bullshit to do the right thing, nothing would ever happen. Making women and young girls feel insecure about their appearance equals money in the advertising companies' pockets. So, it's up to us.

You know the saying, 'Be the change you want to be in the world'. Well the time is now for us to start creating that change. How do we do it? With our spending power! If we all started to vote with our money and refused to buy products from unethical companies, we could as a society begin to show that we won't accept this anymore. We have more influence than we realise, we just need to come together and exercise it collectively to actually make a difference. That's why I am incredibly excited about the Embrace documentary, people have given me a voice and now I intend to flex my power for the future of our children, rather than with the intention of making money or stimulating sales.

One of the first things on my 'to do' list, apart from challenging advertisers about their lack of morals is tackling the issue of body diversity in advertising campaigns, or, more to the point, the lack of diversity. Have you been to a catwalk fashion show recently? No, neither have I, but I have seen the publicity photographs. WHAT IS GOING ON WITH THE MODELS? Are they all sisters? Why do they look the same? Why are so many of them emaciated?

Please, if you are naturally slender, don't think this is about thin bashing, I've seen enough of that in my time and it's just as offensive as fat bashing. My issue with the fashion industry is the lack of diversity in body shape of the models. Just Google 'fashion catwalk models' and you'll see what I mean. Mostly tall and thin is what you'll notice. But here is the paradox, fashion designers are selling clothes to us, and we come in all shapes and sizes, so why is only one type of body used to represent the broader market of the wide, short, thin, lumpy, bumpy, curvy women that make up the shopping public?

When I was being interviewed on TV recently, I walked in the green room and ran in to none other than Mr Alex Perry, one of Australia's most well known fashion designers. Inside my head I was like 'bingo', I was so excited to have the opportunity to talk to him (and, I thought, basically tear him apart).

Alex had recently come under fire for allowing a girl that was severely emaciated to walk down the runway wearing his clothes. The story was headline news across the country. When I asked Alex about his reaction to this, the first thing that struck me about him was how genuinely troubled he was. I had always pegged him as being a bit of knob, wearing his sunnies on his head and all, but he was completely likeable and nice. Dammit! We only had the opportunity to talk for a few minutes but basically he said that this was an industry-wide problem, and that everyone needed to be part of the solution. 'You can't only say designers shouldn't book those models... You know what, let's say model agencies shouldn't recruit those models, magazines shouldn't shoot those models.'

I understood what he was getting it, basically they all played their part in the problem, and they were all in it together. It got me thinking, how could the cycle be broken? It would take a visionary, a true leader within the industry to stand up and lead the charge and create the change. I think if that person existed we would've seen some change by now after all this is not a new problem, it has been going on for years. So, as mentioned many times, the change will need to be created by us and the first thing we need to spend some time doing is getting media literate and savvy to the intentions of the big brands.

Let's take Dove as an example. If I had a dollar for all the times someone said to me I should be working with Dove, I'd be writing this book from an island paradise! Honestly, every time I hear those words, it serves to reminds me how far I have to go in educating people that not all is as it seems.

In my opinion there is nothing more transparent than what Unilever, the multinational company that owns Dove, are trying to achieve. They are not in the business of boosting a woman's self-esteem or supporting body and age diversity, they are in the business of making money. Period. I think that the last place that young girls and woman should be looking for advice on self esteem is a 'beauty/cosmetic' company.

I think Dove is a beauty-peddling wolf in the guise of self-esteem promotion. I also think that the Dove self-esteem programs are a contemptuous attempt at getting product placement into young girls' lives as early as possible. Genius from a marketing perspective, but very distasteful if, like me, you think their actions are part of an advertising conspiracy that is having a negative effect on the next generation. There is bullshit all around, and my intention on writing and speaking about it, is for you to look at things differently. When mature women, and mothers, have a handle on some of the issues I've raised here, then we will be able to impart that knowledge on to our young girls, because as God only knows, our girls need some strong allies to get them through the barrage of material that is telling them they are not good enough.

CHAPTER FOURTEEN

Anti-ageing

LAST YEAR MY PARENTS TOOK my family and my sister's family on a holiday to Disneyland. There were eleven of us in total, it was undoubtedly the trip of a lifetime and many beautiful memories were made. Mum and Dad took us to Disneyland when we were young kids so it was nothing short of spectacular to go back with them again, but this time with seven extras in tow; son-in-laws and the grandkids.

On our stopover in Auckland we had some time to spare before our connecting flight, so we went to the food court to grab some sushi. The duty free shops were just a stone's throw away so Mat and I decided that we would 'tag team' ten minutes each to go shopping.

For anyone reading who hasn't got children the definition of tag teaming when you're a parent is having an allocated amount of time to do whatever you like while the other parent watches the kids. There are a couple of things to keep in mind to ensure a seamless tag team: 1) Synchronise watches and 2) Never be late, always stay within the time frame. It really isn't what you do that is important, but rather the sense of freedom you 'feel' in your free time!

It was my turn first, so armed with a purse I strode long and fast into the duty free shop. Now considering I don't wear perfume (don't do chemicals), don't smoke and very rarely drink or wear makeup, the choice of goods was quite limited, but there was something that caught my eye nonetheless – Brad Pitt! There was a large image of him, modelling for Chanel. The photo was black and white and it was striking, Brad looked devilishly handsome. Once I got past my, 'Ooo hello handsome Brad,' moment, a few steps on I noticed a same-size photo of Linda Evangelista, also posing for Chanel. But there was something very unusual about Linda's face. Huh? This is weird I thought, I knew they were of similar age (and later found out only a year apart) so why does Linda look twenty years younger than Brad?

Linda's face had been completely smoothed out, all of her natural lines had been removed. I stood there for a while going back and forth between Brad and Linda, I am sure I looked quite odd, taking photos and looking around to see if anyone was watching me, the sales staff must have thought I was casing the joint!

After the initial surprise of what I saw, I immediately began to feel the bubbling sensation of anger in the pit of my stomach. 'No Taryn, not now, you are on holidays.' So I parked the emotions and finished up my last few minutes of free time before heading back to tag team Mat.

Nearly fifteen months on and those images still irk me. It's bad enough seeing an image that is heavily photoshopped at the best of times, but to see such a stark difference between two humans similar in age but 'treated' very differently, and modelling FOR THE SAME COMPANY is just deplorable.

Ageing has been dubbed by multibillion dollar industries as a problem that must be solved. Have you seen some of the ads? I mean c'mon, get serious, they are just so laughable. Words like FIGHT, BATTLE, BEAT and TARGET – um, I'm slightly confused, are we fighting a war here or what?

Let's take, 'fight wrinkles,' as an example – why would we do that? It doesn't make sense to fight something that is a natural evolution of the body. Fight 'a disease' I get that, fight against an injustice, sure, but fight against wrinkles, it's not right!

Women! We have been brainwashed into thinking that the natural process of ageing is a personal failing and something to be ashamed of; and of course it's not. I think it's time to put down the wrinkle cream and stop fighting and start loving what we see in the mirror, lines and all.

I have a saying that goes like this: 'The lines on my face serve to remind me that life is short and the bucket list is long'. When I see wrinkles, I think woaaah slow down life, I have so much to do and achieve, not, aggh! I look old and weathered I must go and spend hundreds of dollars fighting the inevitable.

Many of the anti-ageing advertisements shout the message, 'When you have younger skin, you will have it all'. Does this mean they are saying that older women, or women with wrinkles don't? What's wrong with ageing, but more to the point where do all the natural ageing women over fifty go? If the media were to be believed, they seem to disappear!

The next time you go to a shopping centre, take a look around and notice the visual displays – do you see many women over fifty? What about in magazines or presenting programmes on television? Nope don't see too many there either. Where are they? I tell you where they are not, they are rarely found in Hollywood films, that's for sure. Over the past few years I've seen some really bizarre casting of women playing the role of a mother to an unusually similar in age actor. The trend is odd and slightly disturbing too.

Take the movie *Alexander*. Actors Angelina Jolie played the role of Queen Olympias, mother of Alexander the Great, and Colin Farrell played Alexander. At the time Angelina was twenty-eight and Colin was twenty-seven. Huh? Don't you find that very bizarre – why wasn't a more age-appropriate actress cast? Surely it would make more sense if Jodie Foster or Michelle Pfeiffer or... um, I'm struggling to recall more than a handful of female actors in their forties and fifties – funny that.

Where do they all go? What is wrong with women over forty and fifty years of age? Why do they become invisible? Why are older women not qualified to play the role of an older woman? Why is it necessary to bring in a younger version of them? It simply doesn't make sense to me.

And while I'm at it... (starting to feel 'ranty', watch out!) Why are ageing men regarded as distinguished, virile and powerful, while ageing women are considered to look tired and 'old'. Why are the few older women who are on our screens so often injected with poison so that their faces hardly move? AHHHHH, It's complete and utter madness – please tell me you can see it like I do. And if you haven't until this point, can you please join me, there's plenty of room on this side of the fence.

If by any chance you are reading this and you're in your twenties and thirties and think it's not relevant to you, well in the blink of an eye you'll be fifty too and unless we address this issue now you'll experience the 'invisible' dilemma too. Only then you'll feel too insignificant within society and your voice won't be heard anyway. Could you imagine how it would feel to be so overlooked and disregarded?

In a culture that advocates a relentless quest for eternal youth and physical beauty there are going to be casualties. We've seen the very physical results of women in Hollywood succumbing to the pressures to look young, the result being expressionless faces and frozen smiles, and now the casualties are filtering down to you and I, and our daughters. When I was growing up in my teens (and still attempting to grow up in my early twenties) the idea of having surgery or injecting something into my face was virtually unheard of, these days it's as common as going to the dentist. Even the good old Tupperware parties seem to have been replaced with Botox parties and cosmetic enhancement parties!

We need to take a stand now and say, 'No thanks, I don't buy into your bullshit, there is nothing wrong with ageing, I don't need to look younger, I am who I am and I'm exactly as I was meant to be.' We need to be the voice of reason in this crazy world that seems to show so little regard for authenticity. As sure as I know that the sun will go down tonight, no one who is profiting from your insecurities will be getting you to embrace your wrinkles any time soon!

Speaking of embracing wrinkles...

Last year, America's Christie Brinkley was on the cover of *People* magazine with the headline 'Christie at 60!' and a big question, 'She's *How* Old?' Christie was posing in a blue swimsuit, skin and body flawless, looking a similar vintage to me, despite being over twenty years older. Christie's answer to how she looks so good at sixty, wait for it... smiling and fresh air!

I've seen these types of articles before, when celebrities attribute their ageless beauty to drinking water, or playing tennis and ignoring the fact that they've engaged in Botox and cosmetic enhancement and their photo has been photoshopped beyond recognition. It really is a joke, as well as being reckless and highly irresponsible.

Now don't mistake me here, this is not about damming those who engage in surgery and other age defying solutions, this is about the lies that we are told and the bullshit we are fed. If the Christie Brinkley article really was about celebrating her age, then don't you think it's an enormous contradiction to photoshop lines and wrinkles from her face and body? It sounds to me that the article is celebrating fake youth in the guise of celebrating ageing.

I want to see a sixty-year-old woman grace the cover of a magazine who looks sixty and is genuinely embracing her lines and her age. I don't want to see a manufactured 'youthful' version of her, I want the real deal. And I am not alone. I've spoken to tens of thousands of women on this particular subject and the voice is strong – give us REAL images. (And just on a side note, give me real images not 'real women' after all, all women are real.) I get slightly irritated when I see headlines on social media that say 'Real women are curvy', because it's wrong! Skinny women are real too! We are all real!

Why are we only celebrating ageing when someone looks at least twenty years younger than they 'should'. There is a wide gamut of what sixty looks like but to keep using surgery and photoshop as the benchmark doesn't do us women any favours. It sets women up to continually fail to achieve a standard of beauty that is unobtainable. As the saying goes, 'Even the girl in the magazine doesn't look like the girl in the magazine'.

There are some cultures around the world who have got it right, that embrace ageing, and the elders in their community are honoured, celebrated and respected. In South Korea as an example it is customary to have a big celebration to mark someone's sixtieth or seventieth birthday. The *hwan-gap* marks the end of a cycle of a person's life and the beginning of a new cycle. Note, the beginning of a new cycle, not the stage at which you become ignored and banished from society. Maybe I should go live in South Korea!

Speaking of birthdays I love celebrating them (apart from last year when, as you know, I was trimming my beard and buying tea towels). I think that every year we are here on earth and alive should be honoured with a small celebration focused on how grateful we are to be living. How many times have you seen an eye roll or a sigh or just heard the inflection in someone's voice when they say how old they are. Instead of the answer to someone's age being a chirpy forty-seven, it's often an embarrassed or self conscious low-toned forty-seven.

One woman who is definitely embracing her age, is Bridget Sojourner. Now, we all know there's no better place to procrastinate when you are really busy, than on Pinterest. Last year under the pressure of a deadline I was perusing Pinterest and came across a photo of Bridget. The photo stopped me in my tracks. She had grey long hair worn in a high bun wearing a bright orange headband, bright jewellery, blue painted nails and killer sunnies. There was a quote from Bridget that said, 'As a young girl, no one stopped me. I was quite like a lot of young girls. Now, I'm unusual because I'm older. When people started stopping me about my clothes I thought, I've been through feminism, racism, all the prejudices... I'm an activist and ageism is the last bastion.'

I immediately adored this woman, and I now have a photo of her in my office. I just love that she bucked the system of tiresome tradition and conformity. Just because she was in her seventies didn't automatically mean that she was going to wither away, wear beige clothes and cut off her hair. She is walking the streets loud and proud and best of all being her authentically beautiful self, which is a rarity these days.

So what can we do to encourage more women and young girls to love the lines of their face? Here's some ideas to begin:

Ditch the eye creams, lotions and potions you're using to defy age and instead invest that money into your health (yoga classes, a new cookbook), or better still give it to your favourite charity. I promise it will give you a better return on investment.

Change your language: banish 'I'm too old' from your vocabulary. Look at your lines in a different way – every wrinkle tells a story, celebrate them!

Recognise your vital role in the solution of a very large problem: be the change that you want to see in the world. Know that you, just you, just one person CAN make a very big difference. If you continue to 'buy in' to the world of anti-ageing then the world is not going to change. If we all collectively 'opt out' then it will! Wise up and smell the bullshit! Recognise that the companies that are telling you to 'fight and defy' ageing simply want your money. They don't give two hoots about your wrinkles, they don't deserve a cent of your hard earned dollar.

Use some affirmations... repeat after me: 'I have been brainwashed into thinking the lines on my face are ugly when in reality the lines on my face let me know that I am living. Getting old is a privilege denied to many, I will embrace my lines and ageing with the respect and gratitude it deserves.'

And this one: 'I will stop carrying on like a pork chop and shut the effing heck up about the lines on my face! I will not be thinking about the lines on my face when I am dying, so why should I worry about them now? Get on with it pork chop, life is meant for living and loving not battling and fighting!'

If you were an ornament to be looked at then I could appreciate that you would like to defy your age and look shiny and new. But you are not an ornament, this is life and you need to live it. Beginning by learning to love the lines on your face is a really good start.

CHAPTER FIFTEEN

Embrace

ABOUT TWO YEARS AGO WHILE RUNNING my photography business, launching Body Image Movement and juggling the endless demands of three children under five I mentioned to Mat that one day I would like to make a documentary, He just glared at me and said, 'Taryn, I think you have enough on your plate.' And of course he was right, I did not have the time to take on one more extracurricular activity, life was already beyond hectic. 'One day, I'm going to,' I replied, and then I parked the idea in my brain until the middle of last year.

2013 was a very very taxing year for me. I was still shooting family portraits during the week, and weddings at weekends, while working on the Body Image Movement in the evenings. I was flying around the country doing TV interviews, writing eBooks, launching the Developing Daughters Supporting Sons seminars, trying to maintain good health, and juggling the commitments of a family. I knew that this year was going to be the toughest, I knew I just had to get through to December, shoot and edit the last few weddings and then close my photography business. This was not easy to do.

I started Sugar Plum Photography about nine months after Oliver was born. Mat had bought me a Digital SLR for christmas and by February of that year I had registered a business name and I was out there promoting myself as a photographer! It was crazy, I didn't even know how to use the camera properly but one thing I did have was a natural eye for what did and didn't look good, (thank God because I didn't have anything else!) When I wasn't shooting for free, I was shooting for very small cash amounts, just to build up a client list. Looking back at the first year of photographs that I took makes me want to cringe, but I guess everyone has to start somewhere. I then spent the next seven years building my business to a standard I am really proud of, and in the last couple of years of business I had reached the point where I didn't have to advertise, work would come to me. I was earning good money and I had enough of it. Photography was actually easy for me, I could choose my hours, I mostly had lovely clients (when you work purely from referrals you mostly get the same sorts of people), and I knew what I was doing. To walk away from it and into the unknown was really scary.

I had planned to finish the photography at the end of 2013 and focus purely on Body Image Movement. So toward the end of 2013, the thoughts of filming a documentary kept popping back into my head. I felt the time was getting nearer.

In November I was presenting Developing Daughters Supporting Sons and needed someone to film the night so I could use clips from it on the BIM website as a promotional video. I put a call out to my photography friends in a closed group on Facebook: 'Does anyone know a good videographer? I need one urgently for tomorrow night.' And a friend came back with the details of someone called Hugh Fenton. I rang Hugh and he was available, on the phone I joked to him, 'Hey, who knows, if you do a good job of this video, I have an idea for a documentary that I'd love to float with you!' The next night, filled with nerves, (there were more than two hundred people at this talk) I met Hugh and he was delightful. Quietly spoken, gentle and calm – nothing like me, perhaps that's why I liked him, he did a really good job following my filming brief of, 'be like a ninja, I don't want your cameras to put me off speaking.' A week later he sent me the link to the promotional video – he had done a stellar job and the next time we met up I told him about my idea.

I told him that I wanted to make a film that showed my own personal development from hating my body to loving it, and how that mental and emotional adjustment had had such a beneficial effect on just about every other aspect of my life. I also wanted to add to my own story, the experiences and inspiration from other women around the world. As I explained this, I just knew immediately that Hugh was the right person for the project, our values were aligned, he understood what I wanted to achieve, and our intentions were the same; we both wanted to work on a project that could change people's lives. Hugh's business name was Enlightening Films, with the tagline 'Engaging Films That Tell Your Story'. This was going to be perfect, but I wondered how my intense and dogmatic ways were going to work with his gentle spirit.

As it turns out, our differences complimented the needs of the project and while locked up together for a week in a small room editing the trailer, not one cross word was spoken. The one and only time things did get stressful, Hugh turned to me and said, 'Feel like a burrito?' DO I FEEL LIKE A BURRITO? – the man talks my language! It was the perfect working arrangement, we got each other, we worked seamlessly together, it was meant to be.

I still didn't have a title for the documentary, however. Anything that is important I always leave to the last minute, as much as I despise the way it makes me feel physically, I always seem to do my best work under pressure. I went to the Operation Global Change group for ideas.

About six weeks earlier, I had started to feel very anxious about whether or not I could really raise the money needed to make the documentary. $200,000 is a significant sum, it was never going to be easy. I felt overwhelmed at the prospect of doing it alone, so I thought I would ask for some help on the BIM Facebook page. This is what I wrote:

'Can anyone help? I am getting to the very pointy end of a project (soon to be announced) and it is becoming evident to me that I will need some support to get it off the ground.

Have you got one hour to give to the Body Image Movement? If you think you can assist, please search for a group I have just set up called 'Operation Global Change'.

I will provide more details in that group. I will need your one hour of power in May or June of this year. If you 'Like' the Movement, you'll LOVE this project! When you join the group please advise what country you are from so I can ensure I have representation from every country across the world!

Exciting times ahead, as always I couldn't do it without you! x'

Within a few hours over one hundred people had joined the private group. Wow! I have one hundred hours of time, how incredibly powerful. Then within a few days the number of people had reached over one thousand, and eventually we ended up with over two thousand. I had my own small army of people to help me, I didn't feel alone anymore, I had support and it made me feel unstoppable.

It was this group I turned to for help with a name for the documentary, and I got some great suggestions; Breaking Free, Body Love, Unapologetic, Roar, Revivify, Truth, and then I saw Embrace. Someone had written Embrace The Movement, Embrace Our Bodies. It sounded perfect. So, thanks to Heather we had named the documentary. The people, mostly strangers, of Operation Global Change were passionate, dedicated, loyal and hard-working and most donated more like tens of hours rather than just one. They not only pledged, but they told their friends, they shared on social media, they rang journalists, they held fundraising curry nights and afternoon teas. They went above and beyond what I'd initially asked for, and I will always be indebted to these people, my friends.

I had decided to use the sourcing platform Kickstarter to secure funds to make the documentary, and I would use the trailer as the introduction to our campaign. Basically the way that the platform works is that anyone who has an idea can pitch it to the world and in return for their hard-earned money you give the supporter (or 'backer') a reward. A poster, for example, or fridge magnets, stickers etc. The only setback with Kickstarter is that it is all-or-nothing, so for example I had set my goal to raise $200,000 in 55 days. If I raised only $180,000 I would get nothing. To receive the funding you must reach your target. This aspect of Kickstarter gave me many sleepless nights, how much would I strive for, what would be my magic number?

The concept of crowd-funding platforms are simply brilliant. They give anyone who has an idea a voice to share their concept and get it financed without having to 'sell their souls' to the devil. In my travels with BIM, I've been summoned to meetings with global corporations who dangled big gold and diamond encrusted carrots in front of me, thinking I would jump on their train, only to knock it back because their values didn't align. Kickstarter and other similar platforms gives us, the little guys, some power, and I will always be indebted to the creators of such an innovative concept.

I spent months and months endlessly researching what projects succeeded on Kickstarter and which ones didn't, and the reasons why. I looked at the language used, the types of rewards that people liked, the goals that people set and how much over and under in percentage people achieved.

In the end I think I could've applied for a job at Kickstarter, I knew it all, except for one fact: I had overlooked the most important aspect of the entire project, getting the approval for my project to go live. It was the Monday before the Sunday launch, I had faffed around for days, tweaking this and tweaking that, and I finally decided it was time to click the 'Submit to Kickstarter' button. I had read somewhere that it took two to three business days to get your project to be approved, as long it met the guidelines. (which of course mine did). On the Wednesday I started to get a little nervous about why I hadn't heard from anyone, we were running out of time. On the Thursday I woke up in a mad panic, and went on Kickstarter to look around for some 'support' options, and then I saw it, a message sitting in my inbox from two days ago. I had never noticed the little inbox before! Basically the message said that I hadn't complied with some of the guidelines and I needed to make some changes before the project could go live. Changes? There is no time for changes! IT'S DAYS BEFORE THE LAUNCH!!! With the time difference between the U.S. and Australia, it was morning for me but they had closed for the day, so I had to wait until that evening to get in contact. I walked into the bedroom, took one look at Mat and burst into tears, he said, 'Not gone through?' I shook my head.

I remember that Friday night well. We were at a friend's house for dinner and I found it really hard to focus on anything because of the uncertainty. It was like having an out-of-body experience, watching my friends and my kids laughing, drinking, eating, having fun, while I sat there consumed with anxiety. We came home at around 10pm (an outrageously late and wild night for us!) put the kids to bed, then Mat kissed me goodnight, 'Good luck,' he said.

I was so shattered from a week of long hours and lots of stress that I lay on the couch and set my alarm for 11.30pm, one hour's sleep had to be better than none, I thought. At 11.30pm I awoke to the sound of annoying beeping on my phone, it was time to get focused, America was online and I had to make my wrongs right and ensure my campaign went live.

I started emailing the Kickstarter support email address, the emails started out very, let's say 'normal' but by 1am the sheer desperation of my tone was very obvious. When I didn't hear back on the email, I decided to take my harassment to social media. On the Kickstarter website there is a section where it lists all of the people that worked at Kickstarter. In an attempt to get their attention, I individually cut and pasted each person's name from the website to twitter and tweeted them this message: 'Desperate times call for... @kickstarter I need to speak with someone URGENTLY in the next three to four hours'. So there was I was, at 1.30am, cutting and pasting name after name after name; each time feeling just a little more desperate. Failure wasn't an option but eventually after getting blocked from a few people (not surprisingly!) I had to acknowledge that I didn't control this situation and there was nothing more I could do.

At 2.30am my eyes were filled with tears, I just stared at the screen for the longest of times. At 2.36am my email made a PING sound and there was an email from Kickstarter. My project had been accepted.

I woke up extremely tired the next morning, having had only two hours sleep, but I was on cloud nine and positively overwhelmed with joy – the launch would go ahead as planned. That Saturday evening on the strike of midnight, in my favourite green robe I clicked the live button and the campaign had begun, and the trailer I had made with Hugh was up and running. I sat and watched for a few minutes and the first backer came through $200! Woohoo, that's 0.1 per cent of the target, it's a good start.

The next day was Mothers Day, so I enjoyed Eggs Benedict in bed and opening all of the beautiful handmade gifts from my children. I never understood when I was young when my mother would say to me 'I don't need you to buy me anything, just make me a card.' I never got it until I became a mother. There is nothing that I 'need' from my children except their love (and occasionally for them to clean their bloody rooms!!) and a messy handmade card – could there be a more beautiful expression of love?

That day I had to travel to Sydney to get ready for media interviews. Walking through Adelaide airport I felt a sense of sadness at being away from my babies on Mother's Day. Thank goodness for a bit cheer from an unlikely character. I had seen George the security man at Adelaide airport a few times on my travels over the years. He was a gruff looking man, with a bald head, bushy eyebrows and a fierce beard. The security line was long, and as I was taking out my laptop from my bag he looked at me and my 'Embrace the Documentary' t-shirt and at the top of his voice shouted, 'EMBRACE, YES! I saw the trailer on Kickstarter this morning!' I was hugely excited that someone recognised the words on just the first day of the campaign, and replied with an enormous and nervous giggle. George then proceeded to yell out to everyone in the security line that I was 'famous' and that everyone should embrace!

What a great start to my travels, I felt like I was on fire, so when I saw the flight crew walking to the flight gate I felt brazen enough to ask them to wear the t-shirts I had in my bag, the answer YES! So, at 35,000 feet the four flight crew 'embraced' and by the time we landed, nearly half the plane knew about the documentary! At the best of times I am a talker, I love to talk and share, it's my great love. But as a nervous flyer my talking, and the velocity at which it spills out of my mouth can be quite staggering.

Waking up in Sydney the following Monday morning, ready for a day of interviews, I felt incredibly nervous about the money raised – it was sitting on around $8,000 and I had read somewhere that projects that get funded usually get within forty per cent of their target within the first forty-eight hours. I had a long way to go to get to $200,000.

The morning television interview was average to say the very least. I did fine and spoke well, but the host completely got my story wrong. She started by pronouncing my name incorrectly (it happens so much that now it's just irritating) and then she assumed I did my bodybuilding before I had my children, and that I had made the documentary already – gahhhhhh, did you not do your research?

I got my four minutes of interview time and that was that. My one and only decent TV interview and it didn't go so well. I felt despondent and annoyed. Not to worry, I thought, the exclusive print media story was about to be released online, that would get things going. Reading the online story made me go from feeling despondent and annoyed to mad and angry. They too had not done us justice, making the story that was supposed to be about *Embrace* about a story about another woman's body image with *Embrace* as an add on bit at the end.

I sat there and screamed out, 'For fuck's sake, throw me a fricken bone someone.' I tried to reflect on what had happened, was I speaking from the ego, was *Embrace* not as worthy as I thought it was? And then I remembered the guest who followed me on the TV show. He was a comedian from the nineties talking about his new comedy show, he got twice the amount of time as me and sure as shit the interviewers knew what they needed to know about him. Why was my story and *Embrace* not significant?

I sat in the hotel room and thought about where to go from here, the exclusive media coverage that I had worked so hard to get for day one of the campaign had failed, I would never get to my target if this was all I was going to get. What was I going to do? So I contacted media outlets overseas and sure enough *Huffington Post*, one of the world's largest online media outlets was interested in running a story. I was in awe of their reach and their power but instead of approaching them as I normally approach the media with, 'Oh hi, this is what I do, I am extremely passionate, I would love to get my message out rah rah rah' (sweet, endearing and hopeful), I went to Huffington with my angst and frustration from the lacklustre approach to my story from the media here. The conversation from me to *Huffington* basically went like this:

'I have a story, it's a good one, your readers will like it, they will resonate with it, they will share it and IT WILL go viral. Now, I am happy to share my story with Huffington BUT whoever writes the story MUST treat *EMBRACE* with the sensitivity and the RESPECT it deserves. I don't want a fluffy piece, we have a responsibility to get this message out to woman all over the world. I am on a mission to create global change, this is not something I take lightly and nor should *Huffington*.'

With twitching knees and short and shallow breathing I am thinking to myself, 'Are you for real Taryn, this is freaking *Huffington*. Who the hell do you think you are?'

But I am glad I presented it that way, because a delightful writer called Jessica, took everything I said on board and wrote an awesome story on me and *Embrace*. She got it right, she showed it the respect it deserved, and guess what happened? The story was pushed out all over the world. The pledges came in thick and fast, and on day six of the campaign more than $70,000 was pledged to my project. A week later I got an email from one of the Editors from Huffington to advise me that my story was their number one story from the previous week.

I was so very grateful for the *Huffington Post*, as they created a knock-on effect for hundreds of other media outlets. For the next two weeks I spent all of my time being interviewed for newspapers, magazines and TV in more than fifty countries – Germany, Kuwait, Canada, New Zealand, Peru, Brazil, UK, Finland just to name a few. I always knew that body image was a problem that women (and men) had faced all over the world, the outpouring of interest and messages just cemented my thoughts.

At 11.01pm, twelve days after the launch of the campaign I sat in my study nook with hundreds of online friends watching *Embrace* reach the $200,000 target. Un-Believable. I sat there as my family slept, and just cried. I was so relieved, so happy but mostly overwhelmed. The most beautiful part of the campaign was how strangers from every country around the world, had helped me to make the campaign a success. Operation Global Change might sound like an elite and very important division of the secret service, but in reality it was people like you and I from all over the world coming together to make the world a better place.

Creating a documentary with a budget of $200,000 was going to be tight, so with the initial funding target met, and a title selected, it was time to extend our financing. Kickstarter allow you to set a 'stretch target' once the initial campaign is successful, so that people who want to contribute can see there's still money needed, so I set a stretch target of $300,000... and we met that too. While it was running we kicked some serious goals and even got the attention of some Hollywood celebrities. I remember waking up one morning and checking my phone only to see a gazillion messages from people, mostly starting with 'Oh my God'. I knew something had been happening when I was sleeping because the dollars on the Kickstarter page were in overdrive and then I saw a name – Ashton Kutcher. His six-word status update on Facebook said, 'This is good for the world,' and attached a short blog he'd written about *Embrace*. Mat was lying next to me, and I nudged him hard, 'Matty, Matty you'll never guess who just blogged about little old me. ASHTON KUTCHER!' Just for the record, I don't get 'silly' about famous people. They are, after all, just like you and me. My dad taught me from a very early age that we are all the same. He often says, 'We all come in to the world the same and we all leave the same.' So my excitement for the Ashton action was purely about the power of his endorsement. On Kickstarter you're able to see what website the pledges from people were directed from, and at the time of writing, just over $20,000 has come from ASOS – Ashton's blog – pretty powerful stuff.

There were other 'celebrities' that helped the momentum of *Embrace* including Ricki Lake, Perez Hilton, Zooey Deschanel, Amanda de Cadenet and the fabulous Rosie O'Donnell. I actually nearly fell over when Rosie tweeted a message about *Embrace*, she wrote: 'I just backed *Embrace* – the documentary that will create global change – on @Kickstarter.'

I responded @Rosie @Kickstarter Um Hi, wow, thanks! Just between us gals, you've backed a winner, *EMBRACE* is going to change lives for millions of women.

And then she wrote @tarynbrumfitt @kickstarter ummmmm hi – can't wait to see it – keep going...

Holy moly, Rosie O'Donnell, what a legend! I loved that she and others came out of nowhere, not knowing me but willing to put themselves out there to support *Embrace*, just like so many others did right around the world. Now that the campaign has ended I am really excited to be starting the next twelve months of filmmaking, what a ride *Embrace* is going to be.

CHAPTER SIXTEEN

Grandma's last breath

LAST YEAR I WAS IN MELBOURNE when I got a call from Mum to tell me that Grandma had developed a lung infection and would only live for another 24–36 hours. Grandma was 89, and was my dad's mother, she had been living in a nursing home for the past three years and while she had normal signs of ageing in terms of deteriorating health, I almost believed she would live forever. She was such a tough women but although she appeared quite hard on the surface, underneath she was marshmallow, and she had a special soft spot for me.

I adored Grandma, we always had a close bond. I remember as a child having sleepovers at her house, we'd eat salmon sandwiches with copious amounts of vinegar and pepper, and she would let me wear her makeup and try on her jewellery. I loved our special times. So when I received that phone call I felt so incredibly sad that her time was near, I wasn't ready to say goodbye. I called up the airlines and arranged to get on the next available flight, and standing in the airport line waiting to board, tears were streaming down my face. I felt out of control, I wanted an opportunity to say goodbye to her and I wanted to be there when she passed, but I didn't know if I was going to have that opportunity.

When we arrived in Adelaide I ran to the front of the taxi queue screaming, 'My Grandma is dying, I need a taxi!' I sat in the back, breathing heavily, thinking to myself, 'What if I miss her by a few minutes?' 'What if I don't get to say goodbye to her?' and, 'Is she holding on to say goodbye to me?'

Dad met me at the front of the hospital and hugged me hard and I starting sobbing in earnest. I don't really feel comfortable getting upset in front of my family, I am usually the bright funny one not the emotional one. Dad walked me to Grandma's room and I walked in and heard her breathing – very loudly, like she was struggling to take each breath. I took her hand and whispered in her ear that I was there and that I loved her.

Throughout the night Mum, Dad and I took it in turns to hold her hand and watch her. Mum and I analysing each change in her breathing pattern and trying to predict 'the moment'. She made it through the night and the staff were surprised that she did. I agreed that there were moments throughout the night that I thought she was taking her last breath, I would whisper in her ear, 'Grandma I love you, you can go now, go be with Jason, Keith and George.'

My Grandma's life had been difficult in the last twenty years of her life. Losing her son and then her grandson, both of them dying in such tragic and preventable ways, had meant she carried some great burdens, not that she would ever let on.

The nurses had administered some antibiotics overnight and by the next day, Grandma responded with a squeeze to my hand and eventually she opened her eyes up and looked around at each of us.

I spent the next few days at the hospital only going home briefly to shower and change my clothes. A week later, Grandma was showing no signs of improvement but her condition was stable. She wasn't eating or drinking, she was going to die, it was inevitable but we all agreed that the best place for her to be would be back in the nursing home, in the high dependency unit.

I had been by Grandma's side for nearly every minute since I got back from Melbourne. Even when I went to the hospital cafeteria I would run there and back through fear of missing her final moment. It was so important for me to be there for her, just like she had been there for me throughout my life. When she moved back to the nursing home, I couldn't see her on the Friday or the Saturday. Circumstances that were out of my control prevented me from going, mainly my children getting sick, and I felt incredibly anxious. On Sunday morning I woke up early, got dressed and raced up to the nursing home. I had some work to do on my laptop, so I said to Mat that I would spend the day working there, just so I could be around Grandma.

It didn't make any difference to Grandma what I did as I sat in that room, she had been unconscious for nearly a week. Her body looked lifeless except for the occasional and very slow breath in and out. I sat next to her and began to cry. Grandma had not eaten in over a week, she was so gaunt. All her life she had been a strong and solid looking woman and now she was nothing but skin and bones lying in bed, with no teeth and looking very fragile. She didn't look like my Grandma. Again I told her that I loved her and that she should let go.

I sat for a while before speaking to the nurse about how long she thought she had to go. The nurse came in and said that she didn't think it would be today, Grandma still had colour and her breathing was still regulated.

I had been there for about an hour when Dad walked in. He sat on one side of Grandma and I on the other; he told me I could go home and that he'd spend the afternoon there with her. I said I wanted to stay. We talked, we held Grandmas hand and I would often feel her feet – hoping to feel that they were cold, knowing that this is one of the signs that death is near. Lying in this bed lifeless was not how I wanted it to be for Grandma, I wanted her to go. I wanted her to be free.

Dad suggested again that I go home, but I just didn't want to, I felt I just had to be there, so I pulled out my laptop and tried to do some writing. I was tapping away only for about ten minutes when I noticed that Grandma's breaths were getting further apart. I looked at Dad and he had noticed too. I felt her feet again. Were they cold? It was hard to tell. Dad and I watched her face intently, her hands felt cold. I raced out to get a nurse to come and check her. The nurse came back in and I said she thought Grandma was about to go. Dad, the nurse and I watched her. She hadn't taken a breath for about ten seconds, was this it? And then she took a breath. The nurse felt her feet and her hands and pointed out that she had lost her colour. We watched her take another breath, we waited and we waited, but nothing. That was her final breath. Grandma had died. I hugged Dad, both of us sobbing, Dad saying, 'She is in a better place now, she's in no pain.'

Mum arrived about ten minutes later and was so unhappy that she wasn't there for Grandma's final moments. Like me, Mum had been there in the hospital every moment holding her hand, loving her and caring for her. I felt really sad for her and guilty too that I was there and she wasn't.

We sat in the room for about ten minutes just looking at Grandma. As Mum and Dad packed up her belongings, I trimmed Grandma's eyebrows. It may seem a little odd, but over the years when I would go visit Grandma in the nursing home, she would occasionally ask me to trim her bushy eyebrows. So I thought as a final gesture to her, I would trim them for the last time.

I'd never seen someone die before. In the physical sense it is quite unremarkable, one minute she was breathing and the next she wasn't. But on a spiritual level it is breathtaking and heartbreaking at the same time. The honour of watching Grandma pass also confirmed in my own mind that there is an afterlife, and that in some capacity Grandma knew I was there. I also believed that she waited for me and on some level I knew that that day was her final day and that is why I knew I had to stay.

If Grandma had the capacity to think during her final breath, I wonder what that thought was? I often wonder the same about Jason. When he injected the heroin into his vein that final time sitting on a bench in a park, what was his last thought. What was he thinking? What do people think about?

Having read some amazing books on dying and speaking to a couple of people in their final days, one of the most common regrets of those on their deathbed is the wish that they had lived the life that they wanted to live rather than the life that others expected them to. Don't you think it's sad that the person dying and the loved ones watching are experiencing emotions of regret in those final stages? It really emphasises the point that I talk about endlessly, which is to be exactly who you are meant to be and to do the things YOU want to do.

So many women spend enormous amounts of their living years consumed by thoughts of their bodies and body dissatisfaction. I often ask women when I'm presenting at seminars, 'What will you be thinking about when you take your final breath?' Can I tell you what I've never heard? I've never heard anyone respond with 'My cellulite', 'My fat thighs', 'My jiggly bottom', 'My big ears', 'My varicose veins', 'My stretch marks'. NO ONE. EVER.

So why do we waste our lives thinking about the things that clearly aren't really that important to us? Have you ever considered what you WILL be thinking about? It's not a thought that most people would naturally be enthusiastic to explore. After all, thinking about our last breath on Earth might just make you feel a little uneasy. But when I've encouraged people to think about this question they often have an epiphany of sorts that is the beginning of a better life, one with more perspective and gratitude.

When I fast forward to my final breath and wonder what I will be thinking, I can imagine it will be filled with thoughts about my children, Mat, my family, my friends, my 'sparkle' experiences, the times we've laughed, giving birth, all the joy and all the joyous moments I've experienced in my life. So using that knowledge, I try really hard to live in that headspace every day. I am sure it drives those closest to me a little bonkers, I know it grates on my mum and Mat a bit! They'll often say, 'Don't you care about...' (insert whatever has just happened, like ding on the car, rip in some clothes, smashed glass etc.) I do care but I don't – if you know what I mean.

Just because I try and adopt this way of thinking doesn't mean that I am immune to getting frustrated by things from time to time. Just this morning I put the cover on the duvet the wrong way around and only noticed it once I'd made the entire bed, I let out a big sigh but then quickly adjusted my internal thoughts and told myself, 'Hey, at least you have a bed to make incorrectly!'

Walking through life side by side with death has enabled me to live a richer and more fulfilling life. What will you be thinking about when you take your final breath?

CHAPTER SEVENTEEN

Motherfuckerhood

MY PERSONAL LIFE IS... HMMM... let's see, how do I put this... CRAZY! Like most families, among the five of us we always seem to be juggling about eight thousand balls in the air at the same time. People always told me when my children were little, 'Just you wait until they are older, it gets busier!' At the time I scoffed, thinking – are you serious? I have three children under three – LOOK AT ME!!! LOOK AT MEEEE!!! But as the kids approach eight, six and five years old, I now understand what people were getting at.

Those first three years were a blur of endless breastfeeding, nappy changing, toilet training and pretending to really enjoy sitting around in a circle singing nursery rhymes. Don't get me wrong I really did enjoy most of the kids activities over the years but those circle times at Kinder gym really killed me, mostly because it was one of the few activities I did with all three of them.

I was often the mother that other mothers would pat on the back and say, 'Oh wow you've got your hands full.' In fact anytime I would take all three of them out together, I would get complete strangers saying that to me. Only just last week I was in the supermarket and a man, similar age to me smiled at me and said those words, I replied, 'This is nothing, the other three are in the car.' His faced dropped, 'I'm joking!' I said. Then we had this moment of awkward silence before I said, 'Okay, enjoy your shop.' Awkward human beings connecting, so funny. So similar to those moments when you go to kiss someone but they go to hug and then you end up kissing their neck. I hate those moments.

Just for the record in case we meet, I am a kisser and then a big hugger – okay?

Speaking of awkward moments with the children, when Cruz was about two, I decided that I would take him to 'Music Time' – a dancing and singing class for toddlers. We went for one class and I never went back, the shame was just too much. My darling Cruz was a biter. If anyone messed with him and he got frustrated he would just bite. It was only a phase, thank goodness, but unbeknown to me his penchant for biting must have reached its peak the day we started Music Time. There were five other mums at Music Time and we all did the predictable introductions of who we were and our children's names before we started the slightly uneasy singing-in-a-small-group thing. Singing in a big group of people is easy but when there are just six of you, it's really hard to strike the right balance when it comes to volume. I never know whether I'm singing too soft and therefore coming across disinterested, or if I'm going too hard and ruffling the feathers of the teacher. It's no easy gig this group participation thing. It was real airy fairy singing too, both Cruz and I were itching to get to the drums and the maracas, but first we had to sing about sheep, sleep and things falling down hills. I'm not sure if it was Cruz's frustration, or if he picked up on my embarrassment at the whole thing, but out of nowhere Cruz glanced at the girl next to him, lunged, and bit her arm. I was so apologetic to the mum, who was delightful and, thankfully, very understanding. A few minutes later when we were travelling around in a circle going on our butterfly adventure, Cruz bit another little girl. SHIT, there is no recovering from back-to-back bites. If I thought that was bad, it then happened a third time, I was nearly in tears, I felt terrible. For anyone that has had a bitey child of their own, you'll probably agree that you'd rather your child be on the receiving end of a bite rather than being the biter. There is just too much guilt associated with being the owner of a biter.

I had to quarantine Cruz for the rest of the session, I had to hold him and ensure that his little chompers didn't go near any other child. The end of the session was near, I just wanted to get the truck out of there, we were under strict surveillance and I felt like the world's worst mother. At the end of session we had circle time and honest to God Cruz was sitting right next to me and I turned my head for only just a split second, and like a Brazilian jujitsu MMA fighter, in one lightening fast move, Cruz mounted another girl and took a bite before I leapt on top of him and peeled him off. I am not joking, this move was like a move from the mixed martial arts octagon. The worst thing was, this time he drew blood. I apologised profusely, said sorry to all the other mums and left. And never went back.

Cruz's biting phase only lasted a short time, but I dare say that he got in as many bites as a child who went through the phase for three times as long. The thing about Cruz is to look at him you would think he was an angel. He has the biggest and deepest blue eyes and when I look at him I almost feel like I could fall into them. He is nothing short of divine... just not on that day at Music Time.

Having three children under three and a half may have been challenging, but it did also have its perks. Because they were so close in age they often enjoyed doing the same things. An annual membership to the Adelaide Zoo was a hugely successful investment of my money, I would literally go to the zoo at least once every single week – even if we only had half an hour to fill.

I really love being a mum, and I adore my children, but as any parent would know, it is often not easy and we don't always make the right decisions, or say and do the right thing. But we seem to live in a world that portrays our world as full of unicorns, rainbow and mocha decaf soy lattes. If I see one more celebrity looking perfectly slim with no bags under her eyes and perfectly styled hair splashed across the cover of a magazine declaring that motherhood is 'bliss', I'll just scream!

I don't think that I've EVER heard one of my friends describe motherhood as bliss – because it's just not! It is one of the best things I've ever done and I smooch my kids all day long and tell them I love them so much that my heart will burst, but a lot of the time being a mum is hard hard work.

And if motherhood wasn't challenging enough, we mothers of

young children seem to get way too caught up with guilt. I was no different until I started changing my ways earlier this year and it has made such a positive impact on my life. Farewell guilt I said, you suck and I don't want or need you in my life ever again! With the challenges of working around the clock in 2012 and 2013 getting the Body Image Movement up and running, things weren't exactly running like clockwork in our house. People would often say to me, 'I don't know how you do it' and most of the time I felt like responding, 'I don't, today's list of failures have been X Y and Z.'

I was sure I was the world's worst mother when I arrived at the kindy for Cruz's end of term show last year at 11.30am. Half an hour after it had started. All the other parents were there with their cameras and video cameras, some grandparents too, and I had missed the entire thing. What made me feel even more guilty was that I lied to Cruz. When he asked me why I wasn't at the concert, I responded, 'Oh honey, I was at the concert, I was just right at the back, didn't you see me?' Thankfully I was able to back up my lie with some proof. As I walked into the kindy doors I hissed to a friend of mine, 'Give me the name of one song they sang.' She replied 'The Pirate song.' So when Cruz looked at me with his gorgeous blue eyes, my heart almost melted when I said, 'You were spectacular in the pirate song, that was my favourite.'

I beat myself up for the longest time after that day, and felt so incredibly guilty. What sort of mother misses her child's kindy concert? What sort of mother has to wash the laundry three times in a row because she has allowed them to dry in the basket three times before hanging them out? What sort of mother forgets to take the school swimming bag to school during swim vacation week? What sort of mother allows her kids to play on iPads because it suits her to have some down time?

I tell you who – a normal bloody mother!

It's just that we often think we're alone in the fail stakes, it's not like we have conversations with other people about their flaws. It's not like you walk through the school asking other mums what part of their day they've messed up. The assumption is that everyone else has their life seamlessly intact while you are the only one just

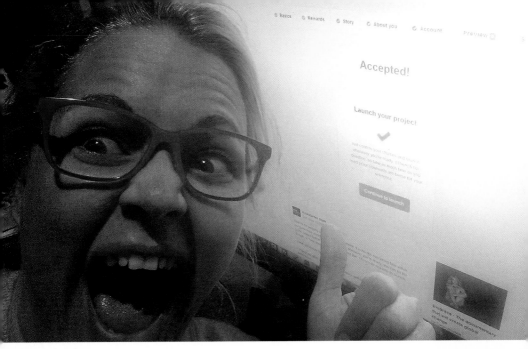

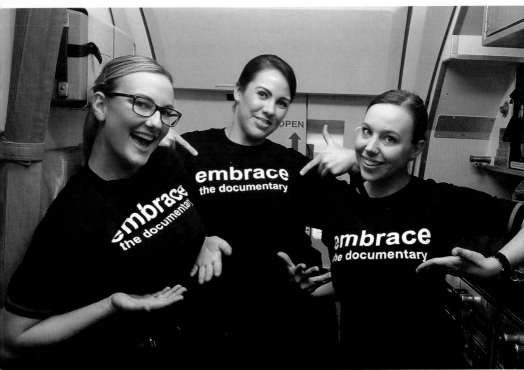

ABOVE: 2.36am Embrace the documentary ACCEPTED just under 24 hours from the launch.

BELOW: Airline crew wearing Embrace t-shirts on Day One of the Embrace campaign... they had nowhere to run at 35,000 feet!

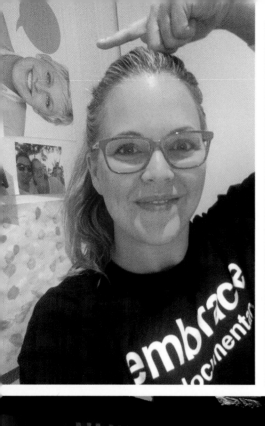

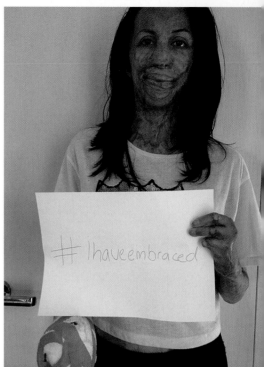

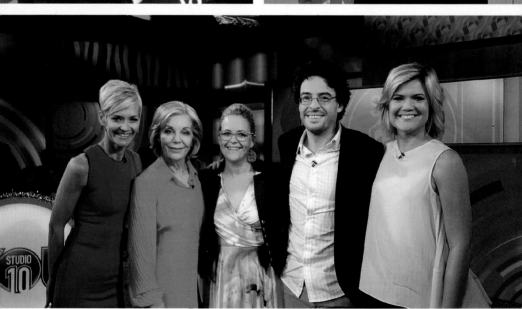

CLOCKWISE FROM TOP LEFT: Interviewing for Huffington Post Live. I was asked to move Ellen's photo from its original position, I guess having her stuck to my forehead might have been a little distracting!; the inspiring Turia Pitt during the #ihaveembraced campaign. The world can learn a lot from this humble, dynamic, resilient and beautiful human being; on the set of Studio 10. I was told 2 minutes before I went on that I would have to 'walk' onto the set whilst being filmed, 'I can't walk on TV' I exclaimed in my nervous manner. I did and I didn't fall over!

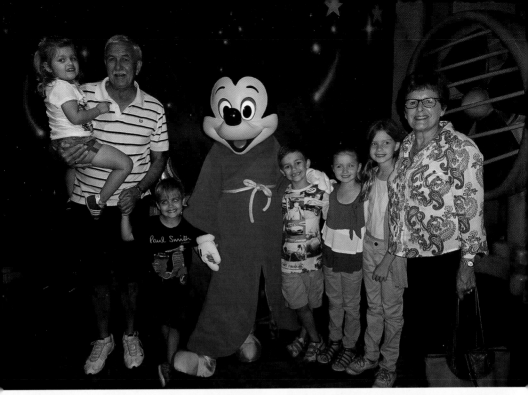

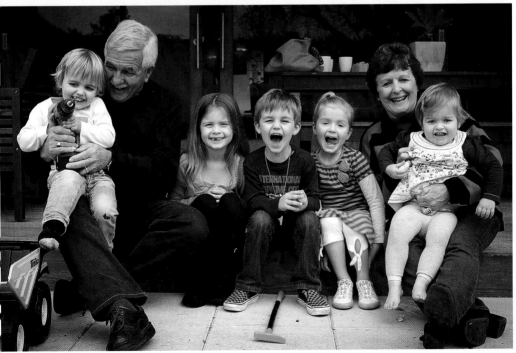

ABOVE: Disneyland 2013, holiday of a lifetime thanks to the generosity of Mum and Dad.

BELOW: My mum and dad with their grandchildren… never a dull moment!

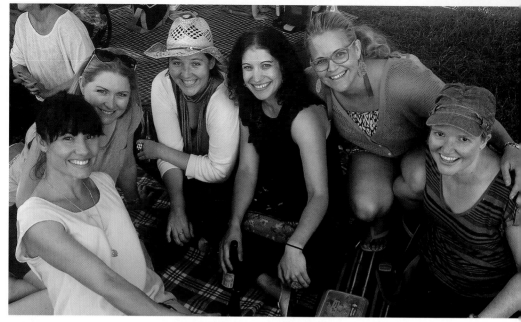

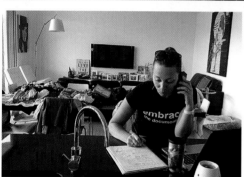

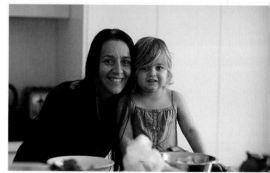

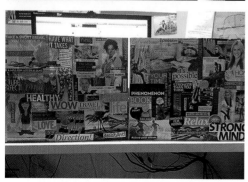

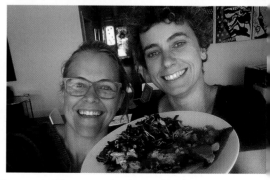

CLOCKWISE FROM TOP LEFT: Danielle, Kellie, Fiona, Kim, me and Emma – school mum friends on Sports Day. I really must stop referring to them as 'school mum friends' and rather just 'friends'; Kelley McPhee aka Aunty Kelley and Mikaela aka Miki Moo; meetings with Dr Emma Johnston always revolve around Emma's amazing leftovers; my 2014 Vision boards and my very messy and 'cordy' office; Martine working from 'our office'. Yes that is all of my washing on the dining room table!

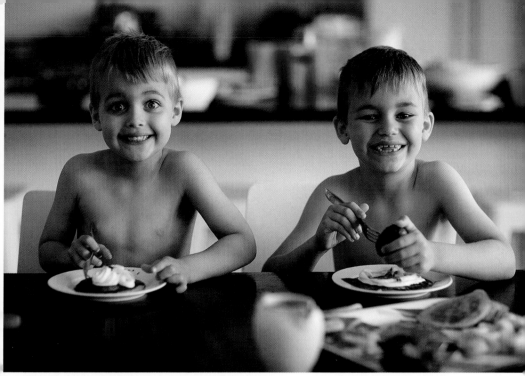

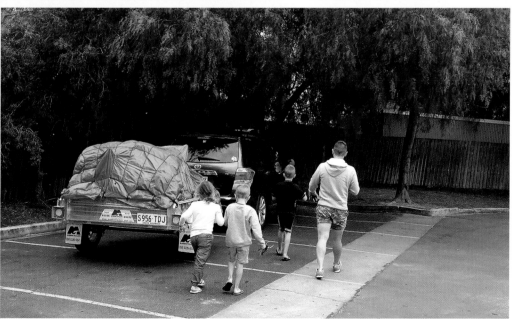

ABOVE: Cruz and Oliver eating our traditional pancakes on Saturday morning.

BELOW: I adore this photo. There's nothing extrodinary about it, but to me it has lots of significance. It's just my crew, on our way camping and stopping for a toilet break.

OVERLEAF: My awesome family and one giant gap in Ollie's teeth from his first missing tooth!

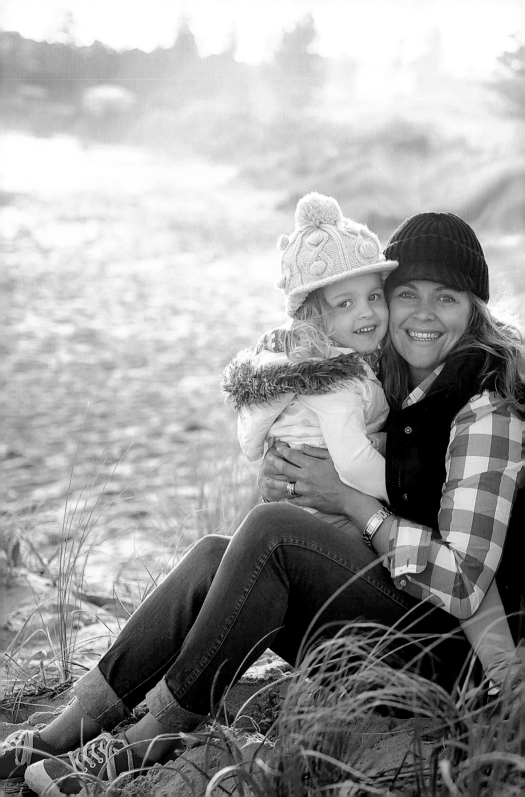

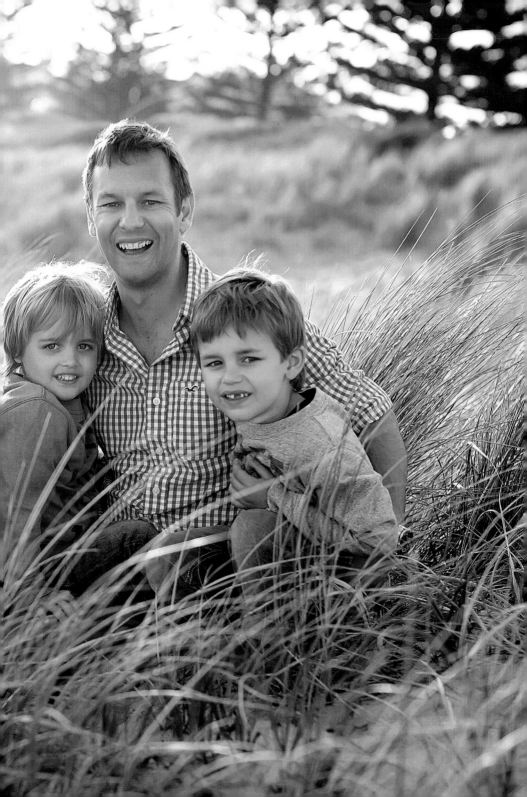

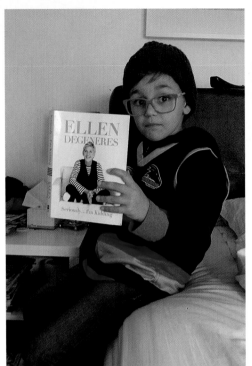

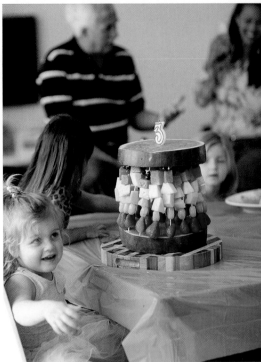

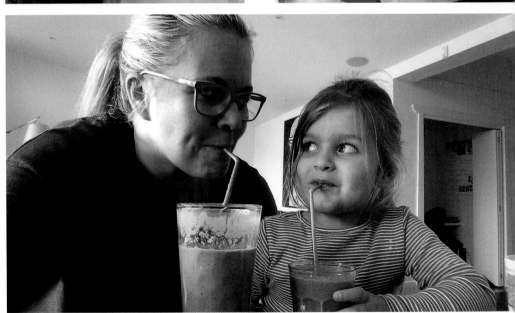

CLOCKWISE FROM TOP LEFT: My eldest son Oliver, 7 years old playing funny buggers with my glasses and Ellen; Miki's birthday cake, love breaking the rules; Miki and I drinking our daily green smoothie!

keeping your head above water keeping up with the endless demands.

The time I forgot the swimming bathers during school swimming week I realised when we got to school, so I rushed home, grabbed a pair of board shorts and went back to Cruz's class. When I handed them to his teacher she said, 'Don't worry there are five other children who don't have their bathers!' Woohoo! Hallelujah! I am not alone! Fist punching the air I asked the bemused teacher, 'There are other mothers out there, doing an average job of juggling a hundred things?! So I sped back home again, trawled through my kids' very untidy (and in need of a throw out) drawers and found five sets of bathers and bounced back into the classroom with the look of, 'I am a rock star,' and saved the day for five children whose mothers had yet to realise they'd no swimwear.

Winner winner chicken dinner! Now where is my mother of the year medal? But of course I had no time to find it, because when I looked down at my watch I realised I was late for Mikaela's swimming lesson! Dammit! Mummy failure! This parenting gig is like an emotional roller coaster – I almost feel like I'm bouncing from a high to a low all day long. It is comforting to know though, that I am not alone. That others experience the same shortfalls as me, five sets of parents leaving home without the swimwear was proof of that.

I think the other unhelpful thing that we parents regularly is compare ourselves unfavourably to others. And just like Steve Furtick once said: 'The reason we struggle with insecurity is because we compare our behind-the-scenes with everyone else's highlight reel.' Oh how true is that?! We often overestimate and overvalue what someone else has, or is doing, and this is no good for our own sense of wellbeing. Imagine if there was a mother and father looking out their window the night that I pooed my pants. Imagine if they saw me running down the street, with my newborn baby in the bugaboo pram, straightened hair and animal print shoes, I'm sure they would've made the assumption that I was in Mummy heaven, looking good and having the energy to run around the streets on a Saturday night! Little did they know!

You just never, never know what goes on behind closed doors!

There is a mum that lives on my street who for years I've watched shine in the role of 'perfect Mummy'. She and her kids are always dressed immaculately, she's often taking them to the park and having tea parties on the front lawn of her house, honestly you would think that this woman was a saint. For a long time I compared her life to mine and often found myself benchmarking my parental skills to hers. I was the mum with the slightly greasy hair disguised under a headband, always running around like a headless chook with children in tow that looked slightly dishevelled. I was doing my best, but compared to her I felt like a failure.

Then one day we were going for a walk around the block with Cruz and Mikaela in the double pram, Oliver piggybacking on my back and Ammo, our schnauzer, on a lead. I was a sight for sore eyes! I walked past her house and I heard her going off her tree at her little one, she even swore. I pretended to stop for Ammo to wee but really I was just standing there in awe, not wanting to miss the perfect mum losing it! Fist punching and multiple high fives all round, the saint is not a saint and I am back in the game!

But what game? Motherhood is not a competition but that's exactly how it felt in those early days when I often compared myself to others and as a result always felt like I was pulling up short of my own expectations.

Since then I've learnt the joy of not giving a rat's arse about what anyone else thinks of my parenting, or me. I know that I am a good person, and I love my children deeply and that's all that matters. I am simply doing my best with my own set of unique circumstances. I've learnt that just because someone has something that I don't it doesn't make them better than me or luckier than me. After all we are all different and it's our differences that make us unique.

But equal and mothers don't belong in the same sentence. There is no equal for mothers, each of us is a stand-alone breed, there is no other like us that walks the earth! In homage to mothers everywhere I am sending you all a cyber trophy – you deserve it!

CHAPTER EIGHTEEN

---

self help 101

SO IN WRITING THIS BOOK it was my absolute intention to steer clear of it being 'self helpy' in any way shape or form. However, having just asked a large group of the BIM followers what they would like to read if I were to 'hypothetically' write a book, they mostly all answered the same – tell us how you learned to love your body.

So I do want to share with you – at the very least – my Top Ten approach and provide you with a list of some of my essential 'things' I do to ensure a high level of body lovin' at all times.

HAVE A LAUGH!

One day I was on the phone to my girlfriend Karen and we were talking about our bodies. I mentioned to her that I could pick my boobs up like dirty tissues, she replied, 'Well, my boobs hang down to my knees, in winter I could wrap them up and use them as a scarf.' Both of us just burst out laughing, it was so delightful to be able to have a little chuckle at our bodies and how much they had changed over the years. People tend to take life too seriously, every now and again it's healthy to have a laugh, especially when it is at your own expense!

SPEND YOUR MONEY WISELY AND GET A GOOD RETURN ON INVESTMENT

See things for what they really are. Just between us gals the companies that are selling you eye cream don't care two hoots about the wrinkles on your eyes. They want your money in their pocket, that's it, the end. The companies that are selling 'feminine fresh' wipes for your vaginas, they too just want your money. And your vagina is far better off without any chemical laden wipe smeared all over it.

Women invest a lot of money into beauty products that's for sure and I did too at one time. But when I began to treat my body like it was a vehicle rather than an ornament my priorities started to change, and the money I invested in 'beauty' was soon replaced by an investment into health products and educational courses that fed my soul. I promise you that investing your money in massages, yoga classes, dance classes, aromatherapy oils and great music will give you more return than smearing some 'miracle' cream on your body!

WALK AROUND NAKED

Get nude! I walk around my house nude as often as I can – weather permitting. I'm not a nudist per se (I do know a few though and they speak very highly of the naturist way of life) but I love the sense of freedom and liberation that comes from being at one with my naked body. I think it is also really good for my children to see that I am comfortable with my body, and it allows them to ask questions about the differences between their bodies and mine, I get ones like, 'Mummy, why is your tummy so big?' I answer, 'Well that's because you guys grew in there and you stretched Mummy, all the way out here!' (Motioning to a big round belly that once was.) They love stories about when they were in my tummy. I also often get questions about my vagina. 'Mum why have you got hair there?' To which I answer, 'Well my darling, around the time you become a teenager your body starts to change into an adult, and adults have hair, some more than others, hair under the arms, hair on the legs, it's just part of being a human!'

If getting nude isn't something you normally do around the house, I challenge you to go hang out a basket of clothes on the washing line NUDE. Just do it, it will sure add a bit of sparkle to the regular chore routine!

DO SOME PEOPLE GARDENING

I've had many people come in and out of my life, I love the saying, 'Friends for a reason for a season.' It's just so true that different people enrich your life at different times, and for varying reasons. There is something that I've very consciously done over the past few years and that is weed out the bad flowers in my friendship garden. I'm sure you could think of a friend or two that has been negative towards you or your new venture, the one who always has a comment, remark or eye roll. It sounds really terrible, but unless there is a really good reason to keep them in your life, get them out of your life. Negativity breeds negativity, and if you are going through a positive change (transformation if you will) then the last thing you need is someone that isn't wholeheartedly on your side.

In the last couple of years I've focused on investing my time into friendships that are based purely on a connection, love and admiration, life has never been sweeter and my garden is flourishing.

BELIEVE IN YOURSELF

For such a long time what held me back from loving my body and loving who I was, was the lack of belief I had in myself. The minute I discovered an inkling of self-belief was the day that I found hope. When I believed I could change, I felt there was hope for my future. So what got me to that point of self-belief, you ask? It didn't happen with a lightning bolt and it certainly didn't happen overnight, it started slowly and I built it up over time, like a muscle. I would like to think that I've shared enough of me, and my inner dialogue for you to have a true appreciation of how bad my body image issues were. And now you see I am where I am. I hope that in some way you might be able to draw some courage from my story, and know that you are not alone in this battle, we've all got our own crap going on in our lives but we also all wield the power to create great change.

FUCK IT, JUST DO IT.

I am definitely going to be getting a word from my mum about the language used in my book, but there is no better way to describe what we occasionally need to do to get a job done, sometimes we just gotta say, 'fuck it' and just do it. Fear of failure will hold you back, the voice in your head that says, 'You can't run 5km,' or 'You won't get that job,' but you can, you might, you will! I cannot tell you how many times someone said to me, 'Oh that will never happen.' Or, 'You really think you can do that?' You just cannot allow lack of belief or insight to hold you back, you are more capable than you know. I would make one suggestion when it comes to learning how to fuck it, just do it, and that is to build up your resilience slowly, don't go out hard and commit to running a marathon straight up, begin by taking on small challenges, get some wins on the board, build a foundation of strength and before too long you'll be crossing that finish line.

TIME IS NOT ON YOUR SIDE, YOU ARE DYING, GET ON WITH IT!

I don't mean to alarm you but while we are living we are all one step closer to dying, so please don't be cocky with your life, get out there and live it. I adore life and I reckon when my gig is up here I'm going to be find it tough to move on, because when you treat life like the gift that it is, it is the most beautiful experience, you never want it to end! One of the hardest parts of leaving Christchurch when Jason died was leaving a life that I had loved. But once I'd done it I felt almost if the chapter had closed. What I was most grateful for though was when I was 'living the dream' (my life, my apartment, Chinese take-away and world's largest karaoke machine) I KNEW I was living the dream, so not a second was wasted on taking it for granted.

So as morbid as it sounds, having an acute awareness of your own mortality can have a life-enriching result! So if the shopping trolley dings your car, if you get caught in a traffic jam, or if you flip your pancake so high in the air it sticks to the ceiling – remember what matters and most importantly remember what doesn't matter!

JIMMY WHO?

I was in a hotel room last month and the TV was on. I don't watch much TV at home, at best maybe half an hour a day, so when I'm travelling for work I love nothing more than to eat my breakfast in bed and watch the morning shows. So there was this presenter talking about fashion 'trends' and what 'you' 'should' be wearing this season. It was just a laughable concept for someone to be telling me what I should be wearing so I could 'fit in' and be part fashionable this season. We are not sheep! Why are we being herded into the fashion pen like that? But what's more, WHY are intelligent, witty, clever and smart people following the leader and doing it?

Now don't get me wrong, I enjoy wearing different clothes, in fact I enjoy expressing myself through clothes and wearing bright colours but not because someone told me too, because I chose to! I get when we are young and learning to develop our sense of 'self' that we are often driven to wear certain labels and types of clothes so we can 'fit it' but why are women in droves still driven to 'follow'?

I knew someone once that was BEYOND BUSTING to own a pair of Jimmy Choo shoes, the issue for me wasn't that she wanted to own a pair of Jimmy Choo shoes, it was the fact that she had never worn a pair of Jimmy Choo shoes before. How could she want to wear something that she's never worn? If you love Jimmy Choo shoes because you've got buckets of money and love the way they look and feel – go to it, Jimmy Choo away, but if you are desiring the shoe because you are being told to, or because everyone else is, don't you think that is a slightly sheepish attitude?

Personally I couldn't give a rat's arse if the undercoat of my shoe is red, or if my shirt has a horse on it, I like what I like because I like it! That means that in my wardrobe you might find a 'labelled' garment but you know it will have been purchased on the principle that I was attracted to how it look rather than the meaning of its label.

There is nothing more liberating than being exactly who you are meant to be, I'm so glad I got off the sheep bandwagon, there is great joy to be experienced in being your authentic self.

GREEN SMOOTHY

It just wouldn't seem right to write an entire book and not include a mention of the green smoothy, I am after all a bit of an addict! From a very young age I've had an aversion to eating vegetables, I really don't like the taste of them. Not cauliflower, not broccoli, definitely not peas, and a big thumbs down for Brussels sprouts. So when I was just pushing myself really hard in 2012 and 2013 (working two jobs, juggling three children) I kept getting sick and run down a lot, until... I tried a green smoothy! I had heard health gurus banging on about these smoothies for years and I always thought 'Bleuch, no way'. Then one day I tried one and they were right and I was wrong, and the best part about green smoothies is that you can put all sorts of vegetables in and the taste is disguised by the fruit.

Green smoothies really help with my energy levels and keeps bugs and illness at bay. Go to my website for a simple recipe and start drinking one a day.

DESIGN AND LIVE THE LIFE YOU WANT

I was talking to a friend last month and she said to me, 'I don't want to be a doctor anymore, I'm really stressed, I am sick of seeing sick people, I just want to go work in a café.' So I asked her what was stopping her? Her response was, 'Because I've spent eight years studying to be a doctor, it would be a waste of my time to walk away now.' I said to her, 'If you are not happy with what you are doing then I tell you what will be a waste of your time, the time in your future.' She paused and then gave me a long list of reasons why she couldn't, the conversation went like this:

Her: 'What would people think of me if I did work in a café?'

Me: 'Who cares?'

Her: 'What if I don't like it?'

Me: 'You won't know until you try.'

Her: 'My parents will think I'm crazy!'

Me: 'It's your life, not theirs.'

We ping ponged back and forth, did some trouble shooting and eventually she came to the conclusion that 'if' she really wanted to work in a café she could, there was absolutely nothing stopping her, but working in a café wasn't what she really wanted to do. What she actually wanted was fewer hours, less stress and more time to herself. So we found some strategies for her to be able to achieve that without having to change careers. What I did notice when we were having this conversation was the glimmer of excitement in her eyes that she could, if she wanted to, change her working life. She could in fact do whatever she wanted to do. Watching her face light up was exciting, it was almost like a switch had been flicked. She now understood that her life was designed by her, that she was in control and she could make the choices and not have to conform to society's standards or restraints. This leads me into my next tip...

BREAK THE RULES

Yes please, break the rules, because you can! Just because you have always done something a certain way doesn't mean that that is the right way or the only way. I adopt the 'break the rules' philosophy with food often. 'You should eat at the dinner table with a knife and fork' – booorrring! I often throw a bunch of food on a platter and eat with the children grazing on the back lawn in summer, or eating an Indian meal with your hands for a cultural experience the kids won't forget!

Food is a really 'safe' example of breaking the rules, there are some 'wilder' and more 'reckless' activities you can involve yourself in to break the rules. Like running in the rain – oh the joy that comes from running in the rain. While it's a bit annoying for me because I wear glasses, the times I've spent running in the rain have been so joyous. And if you are lucky you might find a muddy patch and flick mud up the back of your legs, you'll come home looking like you've played a game of footy, but it's fun! Oh so much fun!

HAVE FUN!

When I was about eighteen, one Saturday night a group of my girlfriends and I dressed up as the Spice Girls and went out and hit the town. It was an absolute hoot! We traipsed all over town to all the clubs getting a roaring welcome as we walk through the door. One club had a stage, so when the club 'happened to' play a Spice Girls song, we hopped up on the stage and gave the crowd our best rendition. It was beyond hilarious and one of my most treasured moments from my teens. But somewhere in my twenties, between climbing the corporate ladder and having babies, I mislaid my sense of fun.

One day Mat and I were arguing, and he said to me, 'You used to be so much fun.' Owwwww! That comment hurt, because he was right, I used to be lots of fun. So you know what I do now? It might seem a little crazy, but I schedule in a fun activity in to my week. It might not be adventurous or wild, but it's a moment in my week that I can connect with my sense of humour and my sense of fun. I do things like climb a mountain or go for a swim on a cold day, take my bean bag to the park and lie under a tree soaking in the sun, put some music on in my lounge room and dance like I'm in a club for an hour.

No one regretted having more fun in their week – try it!

PUSH YOURSELF OUTSIDE OF YOUR COMFORT ZONE

A couple of months ago Oliver asked if he could play soccer for the school this year, 'Of course you can!' I said with a smile but internally thinking, 'OH NO! There is no turning back, my weekends with no schedules and nothing to do but relax are officially over. As the season got closer, I noticed there were no notes, fixtures, or communication from the school, and I asked Oliver what was happening with the soccer team. Ollie looked up at me and with great disappointment said, 'There is no coach I don't know if we'll be able to play. No one wanted to coach.' Without giving it a second thought my mouth opened and the following words spilled out, 'Honey, I'll be the coach.' No sooner I had said it than I was thinking, 'What the effing heck did I just say?' but it was too late, Ollie's sparkly eyes got even sparklier and he hugged me and said, 'Awesome!'

Later, when I told Mat what had happened, he pointed out that I knew nothing about soccer, and he was correct, apart from knowing how to kick a ball, I did not have a clue. It's okay, I told him, I'll wing it, but when I rocked up to soccer training and there was twelve eight-year-old boys looking at me intensely as their leader I knew I was well and truly outside of my comfort zone. But rather than being scared or apprehensive about not knowing what to do, I felt invigorated. Knowing I was pushing myself, and dancing in the world of the unknown was awesome. If you're thinking, ease up Taryn, it's just a soccer team, then I challenge you to take on twelve eight year-old boys and train them for an hour. Let me say, coaching these boys was not easy, in fact I hope at the end of the season I don't get given a poxy mug or a box of chocolates, goddamnit I deserve a trophy.

One of the things about soccer is that you can easily get kicked in the shins, in the first training session most kids rocked up without shin pads – as did Oliver, shin pads; what were they? I soon learned, but only after nearly every child had been in tears from being kicked.

Someone told me that coaching the Under 8s soccer squad would be like herding cats. 'Puhhlease,' I thought, 'I can lead, I got this one in the bag'. Suffice it to say they ran all over me that first session, and the worms on the pitch got more of their attention than I did. Did I mention it wasn't easy?

But here is the lesson. When Ollie mentioned that there was no coach, I could've turned around and said, 'Oh no, that's disappointing,' and been secretly glad I didn't have to add another weekend activity into our lives. And I would've missed out on this beautiful opportunity to engage in the arena of the unknown. Instead I'm off the sidelines, I'm on the pitch, doing something I've never done before, and aside from the tears and the distraction of worms, I am having the time of my life doing it.

SOMETIMES YOU JUST GOT TO SAY 'YES I CAN FLY' AND LEARN HOW TO ON THE WAY DOWN!

If you are thinking but what does dressing up like the Spice Girls, dancing in your living room pretending it's a nightclub and coaching a soccer team have to do with loving your body? Well, it has everything to do with it, it is life and I'm living it with an immense appetite!

Why wait for a bad medical diagnosis, or a sudden accident or some kind of tragedy to occur to decide that you are going to wake up and smell the roses. Go out and smell the roses today! Start doing things that you've not done before, learn a new skill, dance like no one is watching... or when someone IS watching. Let go, be free, give your body pleasure inside and out, use it like it's a vehicle, love it for all that it can do! Go and eat life up for breakfast. Do it, do it, do it, and when you hear those words of doubt running around in your head, think of me sitting on your shoulder whispering into your ear, 'fuck it just do it!'

Phew. I hope that wasn't too ranty or self-helpy, but mostly I hope those words bounced off the page and ignited a little fire within. Go get 'em tigers!

CHAPTER NINETEEN

Mat's chapter

DURING THE WRITING OF THIS BOOK, Martine a friend of mine suggested that it might be nice to hear Mat's side of the story. 'Why don't you ask him to write a chapter?' she asked.

'No way,' I replied, 'It won't happen, he's too private, he doesn't like writing, and he is definitely not one for sharing.' But I indulged her, and asked Mat via email if he would answer some questions, PING, I got a response within minutes, 'Good idea,' and a few days later just over four thousand words arrived on my desk. UN-BE-LIEV-ABLE!

The questions were compiled by Emma Johnston, and no I haven't edited or taken out bits, these are Mat's answers, in his words, expressing his feelings... I am floored, grateful and really proud that he opened up, and possibly have fallen in love with him just a little bit more!

How did it feel watching Taryn hate her body? (and knowing that this was the body you loved)

At first I really had no idea what was going on, she kept it to herself quite well to begin with. Taryn absolutely adored being pregnant, she just loved her belly and was constantly holding and rubbing it any chance she got. After the birth, however, I began to notice a change in the way Taryn felt about herself. This manifested itself in a number of ways but the first thing I noticed was her starting to withdraw socially. Up until Oliver's birth we were extremely social, every weekend we had something on and the party usually carried on at our house; we had some wild parties... however, as they say, 'the game was up!' With the addition of a baby things were bound to change, and I think Taryn used this to disguise her lack of enthusiasm to socialise. On the odd occasions that we did go out I vividly recall her constant battle with her wardrobe. It was an emotional roller coaster for her as she went from one outfit to the next, casting them aside in disgust as she became more and more frustrated with her post-baby body. Being a bit of a neat freak this in itself was frustrating to me, watching the ever-increasing pile of clothes on the bedroom floor grow to mountainous proportions, all the while watching the clock tick by, I am also very punctual just to make matters worse.

Taryn adored being a mother and she was as good a mother as a husband could ever wish for. It is hard to describe her love for her children because it is so deep and intense, she would fight fire, move mountains, part seas all for her new baby boy. She loved the connection of breastfeeding, providing for her baby gave her great joy and satisfaction. While all this love for her child was flourishing unfortunately in stark contrast her love for herself was withering away and it was now evident for me to see.

Taryn would use very hurtful words to describe herself; fat, ugly and disgusting were a few of her new favourite adjectives for herself. I am not the most outwardly emotional guy you would ever meet, and all of a sudden my once positive wife was beating herself up badly and I was under pressure to make her see the reality of the situation. Fuck man, this is well out of my league I thought to myself, we have got some much shit going on in our life right now, why is this happening? Why do I have to deal with this on top of everything else? Anyway, after sulking for a while I manned up as best I knew how. I would hold her while she sobbed on my shoulder, I would rub her back and tell her she was beautiful and that I didn't care about the changes in her body. I would tell her she had just given birth to our amazing, beautiful baby boy and that she should be proud of what she had accomplished and not worry about the changes in her body. I meant every single word of it, she was my wife, I loved her dearly, and she had just provided me with my son and heir. I really didn't give a shit that she was carrying a bit of extra weight, or had a few stretch marks where my son had spent nine months kicking and wiggling every chance he got. I married Taryn for the person she was, her humour, her vigour for life, her confidence, her smile.

I tried with all my heart and might to build her self-confidence back up, but it was becoming apparent I was failing miserably. What I began to realise as time went by was that her disdain for her body was starting to erode into the personality traits that made her who she was. It wasn't the stretch marks or extra weight that put our marriage under pressure it was the sadness and lack of self-confidence.

While all this was going on Oliver had turned one, and suddenly we were trying for another baby. I think Taryn's desperate want for another child seemed to curb her (outwardly anyway) desire to brutalise herself with emotional self torture. After being 'on the job' for a few short months we were delighted to find out we were once again expecting a baby. Soon Taryn's tummy began to grow and the deep love for her baby bump flourished once again. This brought a welcomed hiatus from the body hating habits of the past year or so.

Soon enough we were delighted to welcome our second son, Cruz, into the world. A more angelic looking baby I have yet to see, with the largest piercing blue eyes framed by the longest and most beautiful eyelashes, anyway you get the picture, a good looking lad for sure!

Life as we knew it changed once again, two kids can't be that much harder than one right? Wrong!!! Maybe because we were so flat out Taryn didn't seem to quite have the same amount of time to spend looking in the mirror telling herself how horrible she was. Or maybe she did and I was just becoming more used to the new post-baby Taryn.

I think after all the fanfare of baby number two had died down and we settled into life as a family of four,the topic of plastic surgery began to crop up in conversation. We were big fans of the TV show

DR 90210, where an incredibly handsome cosmetic surgeon, Dr. Ray, with obvious pectoral implants, works twenty hours a day turning what appeared to be beautiful girls into even more beautiful girls with the addition of plastic fantastics and other artificial implants, and sometimes even more gruesome procedures. I recall Taryn saying she wanted to go to Beverly Hills to have Dr. Ray do a boob job and tummy tuck. She felt like she knew and trusted Dr. Ray, I mean hell we watched him every Thursday night we were practically best mates, so he was clearly the man for the job... reality TV has a lot to answer for!

I hadn't really given a whole heap of thought to plastic surgery, however it was clear to me there was a growing feeling in Taryn that her body was 'ruined' and this was the only way to save it. I didn't automatically rebel against the idea but I certainly had my reservations, especially after watching the tummy tuck procedure, if you haven't seen it check one out, it is stomach churning.

Well, all that talk went off the table as life had another little surprise in store for us. Oliver was two and a half and Cruz was just six months old when Taryn and I had a night out on the town. The kids were at their grandparents overnight, Taryn was all glammed up and seemed to be feeling good about herself, and I am always keen to get on it and have a fun night out. Well one thing led to another and before you know it we are back home like the old days getting it on, yeah boy! I vividly remember the exact time of contraception as I was just about to... you know... and Taryn said, 'It's okay, I haven't got my cycle back and I'm breast feeding, so go for your life... !' Well that was good enough me, I proceeded without caution!

A few weeks later I remember Taryn saying she thought she was pregnant, to which I replied, 'That's not possible, you haven't got your cycle back and you are still breast feeding!' I couldn't help but think I had heard these words before somewhere! Taryn then showed me the pregnancy test that she had taken. She told me there was a blue line where the blue line was meant to be, she was adamant. However I couldn't make it out and armed with the knowledge that Taryn hadn't got her cycle back and was breast feeding I was adamant she was not. The next day Taryn once again did a test and this time I was well and truly faced with a blue line where the blue line was meant to be. No matter how many times I read the instructions or tried to ignore that line, two things were undeniable: 1) there was a line and 2) Taryn was pregnant!

I won't bore you with the details but you get the picture by now, the bump grew and Taryn loved it! I however was struggling to come to terms with the consequences of my actions. We were about to be faced with three children under three and a half years of age. I am normally a positive guy and take most things as they come, however this was a whole different ball game! I was very busy at work and travelling internationally regularly, plus trying to manage the demands of a wife and two very young kids. How the hell was I going to manage another baby on top of all that!

Throughout the whole pregnancy Taryn was certain we were going to have a baby girl. I desperately wanted it to be a girl, but nevertheless convinced myself another baby boy was coming our way. I was absolutely delighted to be wrong on this occasion as Taryn gave birth to an adorable baby girl we named Mikaela Rae.

I think it was only a couple of months after Mikaela was born that I booked myself into see the urologist for the snip. I now knew that I couldn't be trusted, and with three kids under four the thought of another was too frightening. I decided that being a big man and all that, I wouldn't need to have a general anesthetic for the procedure. Wow did I get that all wrong. I am lying on the operating table with my drawers down, exposed to the world, and in walks a large bearded man wearing white Wellington boots. I thought to myself is it really necessary for him to be wearing Wellingtons, I mean what the hell is he intending to do to me? Unfortunately I was going to be wide awake to find out! And if that wasn't enough, to add insult to the upcoming injury, there just happened to be four female nurses in attendance. Guys, if you are thinking of being brave and having the old boys fixed up under a local, forget it, get knocked out and save yourself the pain, and more importantly the embarrassment!

You are probably thinking where the hell is he going with this? Well the tone had been set, it was time to get things fixed and I had unwittingly set the precedent. The talk of surgery had started to raise its head again. As I mentioned previously I was very apprehensive about Taryn taking this route however I knew she was desperately unhappy with her body and it was impacting on her self esteem in a very negative way. So, I humoured her, and off we went to see the surgeon. He was very matter of fact about the procedures that would be needed to 'fix' Taryn. I remember him talking about cutting out the nipple and then cutting out the excess skin and sewing it back on. I am a little on the squeamish side when it comes that kind of thing, especially when it relates to the woman I love. He went on to talk about the tummy tuck, as I mentioned earlier pretty gnarley stuff. If I was apprehensive about her having this done before that appointment I was a whole load more apprehensive now! I really didn't see why Taryn wanted to have this done, I didn't care about her stretch marks or boobs or tummy so why did she, and why was it so important to her to have this done?

Taryn had made her mind up that this was the way she wanted to go. I realised how important this was to her and selfishly I wanted my old Taz back, I would be lying if I said I hadn't missed her over the past few years! I really didn't want her to go through with these potentially life-threatening procedures, all in the name of vanity, however I realised she was pinning her future happiness on this and who was I to stop her?

How did it make you feel to go to social outings alone?

Where shall I start... angry, frustrated, alone, sad and unhappy, you get the picture! It was not easy to see your once extroverted and social wife go into a dark unhappy place. We were so looking forward to having a family and to be honest Taryn's self loathing put a lot of pressure on our marriage and did take the shine out of the whole adventure to some extent. Life is linear, and to use my favourite expression, 'you live and learn'. I have learnt so much through this process, let me tell you it wasn't easy at the time, however now I know why Taryn felt the way she did. I am beyond happy that she didn't go through with plastic surgery. I never felt comfortable with it and for her to come to terms with herself the way she did was a very courageous and inspirational way to go. And to think we have the most wonderful, adorable little girl to thank for that, God bless you Mikaela, you have been and remain to this day the most amazing blessing a couple could ever receive!

What did you think of Taryn's body during pregnancy, after, and when she was on stage competing?

I loved it during pregnancy, after pregnancy, and when she was on stage competing! You are probably saying yeah right Mat, stop bullshitting and tell the truth mate! Well believe it or not I am! I married her because of the person she is not because of what she looks like. Yeah I know she is hot, so that is easy for me to say right, well whether we like it or not we all age and our bodies change. I know the big cosmetic, fashion and fragrance companies don't want you to accept that because then they can't make a shit load of coin off of you, but sorry it's the truth and the sooner we all accept it the happier we will all be! Taryn went from being pregnant, to being a regular just had a baby mum size, to model thin with an ass you could crack a coconut on (well I didn't actually try that but I reckon I could have), and back again. To me Taryn is much more than the sum of her looks! She is loving, loyal, feisty, caring, courageous, loud-mouthed, a wonderful mother, a great table tennis player, can kick a footy or a soccer ball better than most men, is single minded, annoying, talks too much and is willing to take on the most insurmountable task with an outrageous and unbelievable confidence, conviction and vigour. She is the love of my life, my wife and the mother of my three wonderful children, so to define what I think of her based on what she happens to look like on any given day would be an injustice and for that reason... I simply don't!

Was it hard to support Taryn's decision to have surgery, knowing that you philosophically disagreed with it?

I touched on this earlier and yes it was very hard! People these days seem to think cosmetic surgery is normal, and enter into it with what appears to me as the same kind of blasé manner you might go to the hairdresser with. We have become desensitised to the fact that they put you to sleep and cut you open and put foreign objects in your body. They remove chunks of your skin and sew you back together again and chuck the unwanted bits in the bin. It is surgery and there are all kinds of things that can go wrong. I have no issue with people having it done as long as they have spent the time researching it and weighing up the positive and negatives. But, Taryn is my wife and I didn't want anyone cutting her open and potentially taking her away from her children unless it was absolutely necessary and I definitely felt it wasn't!

How did it make you feel when Taryn decided not to have surgery?

Happy!!!

What was your reaction to the Before and After photos?

I am sure Taryn has mentioned somewhere in this book that I am a quite a private person. So when she posted this picture on Facebook I was pretty shocked! I mean if you polled a group of guys if they would be happy for their wife to put a nude (all be it tasteful) photo on Facebook I think the majority would have been in my camp. What the fuck?!! Taryn thinks sharing everything with everyone is normal; I try to argue that it is not. Have you ever had an argument with a brick wall...? Well you see my dilemma then. I am also not the greatest at talking about how I feel... mmmmm, let's just say I felt like I should have been consulted prior to her doing it. I agree it is her body, however she has a greater responsibility to her family, and in my eyes it could have potentially had a negative impact on her, which in turn has a negative impact on me and the rest of the family. My concerns were valid, however fortunately it had a very different impact, a very very positive one! I mean there were plenty of losers taking pop shots at her with horrible comments. At first I took great offence and wanted to find them and hurt them! But I realised very quickly that these people are just haters and unfortunately 'haters are gonna hate' so now I simply ignore them and focus on the positive and meaningful things people have to say.

What sacrifices do you perceive you and the family have made for The Body Image Movement, and how have you kept positive in the face of those sacrifices?

Well it is has not been a bed of roses that is for sure. Taryn has taken on the mammoth task of trying to create global change on the issue of negative body image. It is a worthwhile cause, and something that is well overdue, so when I am pissed off that I have hardly seen her as she has been held up in the office night after night I just have to remind myself of that. Taryn built a successful photography business, which she gave up to pursue developing the Body Image Movement, I supported this but with it came with some financial pressures. Taryn has worked incredibly hard for little to no financial reward to build BIM into what it is today. I have and will continue to be the support and sounding board that Taryn needs to drive this into the future. There is much work yet still to be done!

What was your initial reaction to Taryn participating in the Sydney Skinny? And since?

Initially I was sceptical and did not like the idea! Some dude contacts Taryn out of the blue to come and be part of his nude swim, yeah good one mate... it ain't happening sunshine! Anyway, as Taryn tends to do, she ground me down and eventually persuaded me that it was a legit event and had a much more spiritual meaning than I had initially thought. I was warming to the idea as I saw the merit in it and more importantly she was beginning to wear me down and often it is just easier to give into her than resist. If memory serves, I think the tipping point was her allowing me to go on another one of my interstate cycling adventures and also allowing me to take the week off for the Tour Down Under. So in short, like most people, I can be bought!! Taryn hasn't stopped raving about the last event and having seen some of the footage I can understand why, she is even trying to get me to participate in the next year's event. I have a fantastic physique (he says bashfully) however I prefer to have it adorned with a light covering of lycra, at least in public anyway!

How hard has it been seeing some of the negative comments about Taryn?

Initially it was very hard. No one likes people saying nasty things about their family, particularly their loved ones. I mean if someone said any of that shit about Taryn to my face that would be it, it would be on like Donkey Kong! Look at your husband and tell me he would do something different... I thought not! Taryn couldn't understand why I would get upset by some of this stuff, she would say, 'Why are you getting upset? It's not you they are talking about?' I had to remind her that I was her husband and that I loved her, it is in my nature to want to protect her. Eventually, like most things, you become immune to some extent, there is no point even acknowledging the negative and nasty comments because if you do you are giving 'them' what they want. I often ponder this subject because I can't get my head around why some people choose to sit in anonymity behind a keyboard and deal in hate. Why would someone do this? What gratification does it give them to slander and belittle good people they have never even met? Asking the big questions now aren't I?! Ultimately you just have to take the good with the bad, fortunately the vast majority of feedback has been overwhelmingly positive and as far as I am concerned the 'trolls' can go and get fucked!

What has it been like to share Taryn with the world?

It was taxing at first but like most things in life you find a groove that works for you and just get on with it. The hardest thing for me has been her obsession with sharing the intimate details of her/our life. I am sure girls shoot the breeze about all manner of things over a cup of coffee, however I have to deal with Taryn making it public knowledge. I tend not to give a shit what most people think of me, however I was concerned about what family and friends might think of all this sharing. I was very reassured to find that the people I care about have embraced what Taryn is trying to achieve and have shown nothing but support. It came a little out of left field when

Taryn asked me to contribute to her book, she thought it would be great for readers to get my insight on all of this. I was reluctant at first however I decided why not! So now I am really stepping out of my comfort zone and sharing some very private details about myself. I suppose Taryn's willingness to share is starting to rub off on me, I will never be the open book that Taryn is but I have quite enjoyed loosening up a little bit.

How important is the Body Image Movement to you?

It is very important to me! I have been there from day one and lived this with Taryn every single step of the way. We have three young children and I don't want to see them put under pressure to confirm to an unrealistic ideal just because it serves the interests of a few. I have seen intimately the impact a negative body image can have on a person and the people around them. Taryn made a choice to love who she is rather than waste her time and energy loathing herself. It is a choice others can make too. If we can help change the way people see themselves from negative to positive then I think we will have made a valuable contribution to society! At the end of the day that is a pretty cool thing, right?

CHAPTER TWENTY

Letters to Taryn

FROM THE MOMENT I STARTED the Body Image Movement I have received thousands of letter, emails and messages from people wanting to share their story.

I extend a heartfelt 'thank you' to all of you, for sharing and for believing in me and in the movement. The following is a selection of the letters I have received.

I put on a pair of bathers, first time in years, and went swimming with my daughter for the first time. She is four and a half, and she was so excited because I had never done that with her before. I am the same size I was years ago, but I knew that what I thought of myself was making me, and my kids miss out on too many things. So it has definitely changed my perception, and I am not afraid of the way I look any more!

Deb Saunders

With a height-challenged father and living on gluten-free diet (which often tends to have too many highly processed alternate grains) my six-year-old daughter has a slightly stockier body than a lot of her female friends. Going through the usual growth phases of out-then up-then out etc. I have never been too worried as she is still within the healthy range. She has however often commented that she 'is fat' after other older girls pointed it out to her in comparison to their body. Having been following BIM from its inception through FB, I have learnt a lot about how to talk to her about the fact we are growing a strong healthy body to carry us through life, not just to be skinny and look good. There has been a lot more focus on how she feels, her health and what her body can do. Thank you for your suggestions, I know they have helped the dialogue in our house about loving what you have. x.

Samantha Griffiths

You finally got through to me! Here you were, this model body builder, and then you were just you and knew what it felt like to be that 'perfect' body and you didn't care, you just wanted to love yourself the way you were. I felt if you could do it, why not me too!

Jennifer Cullis-Mitchell

After having a child in my mid thirties and then a very serious back injury I was carrying extra weight (which I have never done) BIM has proven to me that it REALLY is not about those extra kilos – it's about loving your body through every stage. My body is becoming strong again – I know I will never look like I used to in a bikini but I know I will get into swimmers and get in the pool with my daughter and love it! Keep spreading the message – I know a lot of people that could do with the wakeup call that your exterior is just that... your outside shell.

Ellie Humphris

BIM is an inspiration to so many women. I now look at my caesarean tummy and my breastfeeding boobs with pride – they've done so much! My body is something to love and to be proud of!

Dr Gemma Munro

I love the movement, I love the positive message it sends. As women and girls we need honest, real, positive role models. We need to learn to accept with genuine warmth how lovely we are (with lumps, bumps and imperfections). I want my daughters to grow up and realise how very special, fantastic and individual they are, and love this about themselves.

Kellie Brown

BIM has helped me to realise that I am okay as I am. After 45 years of feeling that my shape is unacceptable, not good enough or 'wrong', I am now learning to undo years of self-loathing that has resulted in neglect and a disconnection of my own body to my sense of self. If only I had BIM in my formative years, the exposure to positive reflections of real women would have helped so much. Thank you Taryn for giving me permission to like my well-worn and life-torn body.

Cha Ka

A few years ago I lost in excess of 35kg and, despite years of hard work to get there, I still wasn't happy with my size. I'm now an 8 on top and 10 on my bottom half. When I saw your photos and started following BIM it gave the kick start to realise that while I was overweight and I have had a child that doesn't mean my body isn't great. I will always have a flabby tummy and tuck shop arms but I am proud of who I am, the life I have had and what lies ahead. BIM really did kick start and continue to reinforce that shift in my psyche. When I stop to think about the negative media around females and their body shape it actually makes me sad. I am so happy you are working so hard to changing those attitudes. I look forward to following BIM's success in the future.

Paula Edwards-Moffat

The BIM has come at a time in my life when I really needed it. I've been larger than I am now, but have realised with your help that my eyes haven't changed a scrap and I still see the same larger me and this has made me miserable. Why? Because of what I've learned through BIM, I've realised just how brainwashed I've been by mags, news etc (in more ways than one) to think that my appearance is not 'normal' & that I'll only ever 'be happy' if I'm thinner or more beautiful. The reality is there is no such thing as 'normal' or 'perfect', and happiness or contentment does not come in the absence of stress, sadness or any of the other emotions we may experience during the course of a single day, let alone a lifetime. Thanks to BIM I am now looking at my face without makeup and not cringing (I think my skin looks better now as a result of more make up free days!) and I'm taking the opportunity to look at myself with a kinder set of eyes... and guess what? Whereas I've always thought 'thunder thighs, too much tummy, batwing arms,' now I'm seeing the lean strong legs that helped me run my first City to Bay 12km last year, my strong arms that allow me to hug my kids, and a soft white tummy that my kids love to lay on or touch, proudly knowing that I carried them there... I've still got a way to go, but the Facebook community you've created and the conversations that have been sparked make me hopeful that my son and daughter will grow up without the image issues their parents have had!

Gabrielle Preston

BIM makes me realise, and really feel, the connection I have to all women. That it doesn't matter why our bodies look the way they do, that it doesn't have to be a competition about who looks the worst or the best, whether you have kids or a partner, whether you are 'working on it' or not. I can lovingly look at my body and pat the wobbly bits and be genuinely glad they are there, as well as wanting good health and increasing my self confidence. Just as I am, just in this moment. LOVE this being in my world.

Claire Latham

I was hating my post-baby body and therefore HATING myself. When I read your story I began to sob. It had never occurred to me to just change my mind, ignore the voices and love my body just the way it is. Not just in spite of but for all the reasons I hated it. The stretch marks proving my stomach grew and held children inside. The fact that it is strong enough to not only carry these children but to birth them! Changed my whole life. Thank you.

Michelle Kaiser Romo

Happy Friday to you too! BIM helped me accept my stretch-marked and saggy tummy as a badge of honour instead of always wishing it was different due to unrealistic magazine articles on buffed abs etc with pics of women who hadn't even had children!! Thanks for making it okay through positive reinforcement and putting yourself out there and showing that we are all unique and not cookie cutter women! X

Sue Dunford

I now feel like I don't have to chase an unrealistic and impossible image. I have stopped looking at twenty-something bodies as peers. I no longer feel repulsive that I too have a smile across my belly from my son's creation.

Elizabeth Leonard

CHAPTER TWENTY ONE

Frequently asked questions

Where do you get all your energy from?

Life! I feel so energised by life! I love life, I love *my* life and the people around me. I feel so incredibly blessed to be living. Feeling like this gives me energy.

From a physical perspective I do strive to fuel my body with lots of goodness.

I do have lots of energy that much is true, BUT you must remember that when I am in public, or speaking, or on interview I am totally buzzing with excitement too, and then feel totally exhausted afterwards.

How can I stop the guilts now I've tried to 'embrace' being healthy and happy with my body but my friends and family assume I have somehow given up instead?

You have NOTHING to be guilty about, so kick any thoughts of remorse or shame to the curb. You have chosen to love your body and what will happen when the love strengthens within you, is that it will RADIATE from you and it will begin to positively affect others.

In the early stages of the 'new you' (!) it might take some friends and family some time to adjust to your new way of thinking, but before too long they will see the joy and the happiness that comes from loving your body from the inside out and they will get on board. (And if they don't, maybe you need to sit them down and explain how you don't like weeds in your beautiful garden!)

How do you deal with your emotions surrounding your stomach now? And do you feel judged by others for not having the surgery? I know there are still many women who see nothing wrong with plastic surgery.

I don't really have any emotions about my stomach, it is after all just my stomach. It's the place that housed my three babies, and it was stretched and therefore has stretch marks. I look at my stomach and my entire body very differently now, I have a new appreciation for it. Here's an example; this morning I ran up and down the soccer pitch at a game coaching the team, I sprinted, strode, walked, and jumped in the air a few times when they got goals. My body allows me to do exactly what it needs to do, I am just grateful. Does it matter that my tummy looks white, lumpy, stretched, saggy? No. What matters is what my body can do! And my body can do everything I want and need it to do!

As for feeling judged by others for not having surgery, no I don't. The only people that I've had comments from on about whether I should've had surgery are the negative trolls – but I don't listen to them anyway!

How do you fit being an activist, mother, wife and friend in? It must be a tough schedule?

At times the schedule is relentless and when the balance is out I don't feel at peace or in a good place. Last month I worked over one hundred hours a week, the pace has been frenetic and the schedule gruelling and to be honest I've not been a good friend or a good wife! I have just managed to protect the children from my schedule, working late and when they are in bed but that has come at a cost to my health.

Striking the right balance is crucial but it's also important to respect that there will be times (like now) when sacrifices need to be made. During the peak times I try to ensure that I am giving my body everything it needs to run like a machine. Putting your body under too much stress will result in fatigue or illness, and that's something that you don't need when you are working to a deadline.

In terms of some of the practical things I do to keep my wheels turning, I try and do several five-minute meditations through the day to refocus my mind, I use lots of essential oils, I drink green smoothies, lots of water and at least once a week I get a massage, which sounds pretty decadent but I think it's a really valuable investment. I don't use creams, lotions, potions, perfume, I rarely drink, I don't have time to shop, so I seldom spend money on myself – I can totally justify a weekly massage!

Where do we draw the line between 'wear what you want' and 'dress to your (post-baby) shape'?

I didn't know there was a line? I say wear exactly what you want and when you want so long as you feel comfortable. Dress for comfort, and dress to make yourself happy, no one else!

How do I encourage my friends to feel beautiful?

Encourage others to see the beauty in their body beyond their appearance. Teach them a new currency for beauty, the one we can't see. Here's a story that you might be able to use to find your own experience to share with your friends.

I have met so many women, and actually I have to include myself among them, who have totally and completely fallen in love with their male obstetrician or gyno, and have gushed about how handsome and attractive he is. And you know what, often there's nothing particularly remarkable about his looks, the reason why they attract such adoring admiration is that they just radiate kindness, compassion and care, and they look after us at one of the most vulnerable points of our lives. When we say that a person like this is incredibly attractive, we are talking about their depth of character, and the beauty within.

On the other hand I have met some women in my time that have been touted in the press as 'most beautiful', but when I've spoken to them, beautiful was the last word that would spring to mind. You can't see beauty, it lies within. It has nothing to do with our appearance.

In society today there is a strong association between being skinny and being healthy. How would you address someone that says the thinner you are the healthier you are without shaming those people who are naturally thin?

It all comes back to 'you cannot judge someone's health by their appearance'. Skinnier, fatter, it doesn't matter what your shape or size, your health is unique to you and is not necessarily determined by the amount of fat or the lack of fat on your body.

I think as a society also we must be mindful that the language we speak to share our positive intentions to 'love our bodies' doesn't alienate or offend another culture or body type.

As an example when I've posted a photograph of a curvy woman, I've seen comments that say things like, 'Yeah men love women with curves, not skin and bones.' Effectively that person is criticising a person who is thin. We must learn to promote body diversity rather than promoting a body type.

Can't you love your body AND want to enhance it with plastic surgery? Who is to say wanting plastic surgery means you don't love your body?

I respect that everyone has the right to make their own choices without judgement from others. What I am trying to do with BIM is give people an alternative to having cosmetic surgery. I want to provide people with the hope and belief that they can love their body without changing it surgically.

It doesn't mean that people who have had physical enhancement don't belong at BIM, we are after all inclusive not exclusive!

How do I learn to love what I see in the mirror?

I think learning to love yourself happens away from the mirror. Self love comes from within as do all the qualities that make a person beautiful. Reflect on the person that you are; are you a kind person, a considerate friend, would you help a stranger in need? If someone was cold would you lend them your jumper, if someone was hungry would you give them a meal, if you saw an injured animal would you stop to help? Humility, kindness and compassion should be the currency of beauty, so that when you look into the mirror the knowledge that you are a 'good person' is totally loveable!

How do you reconcile knowing that you need to lose a couple of kilos to be healthy and loving your body as it is?

Firstly, there is nothing bad about wanting to be the best you can be, however I would recommend your focus remains on health and not your weight. Chasing a number on the scales doesn't define you, your health or your happiness.

My fitness and health ebbs and flows depending on my workload, social calendar and stress levels. In an ideal world I would maintain my health at a consistent level but life doesn't run perfectly smoothly and nor do I! When I am feeling a little 'under' and not performing at my best, I address the issues that are affecting my optimum levels. For example, when I have deadlines to meet, I will often sit at my computer all day and into the night, and in the evenings I eat lots of chocolate. Sitting all day is really bad for my neck and back, and a bi-product of not moving my body and getting out in the fresh air is high levels of grumpiness! I don't need a set of scales to tell me that I need to be moving about some more, my body gives me all the indications I need.

If I did use the scales as an indicator of my wellbeing I am sure they would show an increase in weight. I've stood on the scales plenty of times and it has never been a joyous or particularly motivating occasion. After a period of unhealthy behaviour, however, I do feel inspired to get outside and improve my energy levels, because I want to feel good again.

Do you ever slip back into old patterns of thinking about your body? And if yes, what do you say to yourself to shake that off and renew your commitment to self-acceptance?

This is a great question. No I don't fall back into the really destructive negative patterns, but I have on very rare occasions had a moment of, 'Grrr my clothes don't fit me!' But my frustration has been directed at the size of my clothes not the size of my body! I love and respect my body so much now that I only have nice things to say to her and about her. She has given me so much, I am in awe of her talent, resilience and abilities.

How do you cope with the constant chatter of friends around you who are dieting or talking about diets?

I think because of what I do my friends rarely talk about dieting in front of me! In fact I'd like to think that most of my friends also believe that diets don't work so they don't actually engage in them!

If you have that problem, I would gently suggest to your friends that they do some research on diets. The statistics are mind-blowing, a recent study showed that ninety-five per cent of dieters put the weight back on when they finish the diet, and in one large study, two thirds of participants ended up heavier than they were before dieting. We have more diets on the market than we've ever seen, and yet the population is heavier than it's ever been.

So if not dieting, then what? It comes back to focusing on health and most importantly listening to our intuition. If you've never tapped into your intuition then now might be a good time to, it is an incredibly powerful tool to use in life. For great health our bodies need water, good fresh 'living' food, rest, sunshine, fresh air and our bodies need to move. That's it, really bloody simple – right?! I think the answer to society's health epidemics lies within the individual, not on the branding of another 'revolutionary' and 'transformational' product.

I have a thirteen-year old daughter and I guess my quest for being healthier reads as being unhappy with myself. I recently caught her saying, 'If I eat another bite, I'll become a fatty'...wow!! How do you approach striving for better health without encouraging the next generation in their self-hating beliefs?

Can I assume that the things you are doing to strive for better health are positive things? If so, then explain to your daughter that you want to live life with lots of energy, so you are fuelling your body with good food, or that you move your body because you love how the endorphins exercise produces make you feel.

My friend Emma Johnston took up running last year and when her boys asked her why she was running she replied, 'So I can keep up with you kids!' And then she chased them away, much to their delight! I thought it was a great answer.

Emma's friend Sarah came to her recently for advice about her eight-year-old daughter who had started saying she was fat and needed to go on a diet. Sarah had recently started a 'transformational' diet and fitness challenge at her gym and as she restricted her calorie intake and increased her exercise was beginning to noticeably lose weight, a result that she was delighted about and was quite open in sharing with her family. Friends would also exclaim about how great she was looking. Emma discussed with Sarah the messages her daughter was receiving and how confusing they must be; her mother was eating different food from the rest of the family and spent lots of time at the gym to get rid of 'fat'. In fact, in her daughter's mind this fat must be so bad that even her mum's friends were pleased some of it had gone away. The natural consequence of this was that Sarah's daughter wanted to mimic her mother and get the same approval; she wanted to be on a diet too.

Emma didn't suggest to Sarah that she should abandon her quest for better health, but that she should change the ways she discusses and perceives it; when talking to her daughter and others she could talk in terms of feeling stronger, moving faster, and having more energy, rather than in terms of weight loss or fat reduction.

How do you maintain your beautiful, positive attitude when you have had so much negativity thrown at you?

Strangely enough the negativity actually drives my positive attitude. It makes me want to work harder to get my message out to more people. My story and my vision for people across the globe is so genuine and authentic, and comes from a place of care and love, that I feel completely sure and confident about it. Articulating is difficult, but I feel unshakeable, unbreakable and unstoppable!

I also know that the shit that's dished up is their problem and not mine. Lastly I feel I have the support of millions of people around the world, and that's really comforting to know too!

Do you really believe that you can create global change?

Yes of course otherwise I wouldn't be doing this! The Embrace Kickstarter campaign filled me with lots of confidence, the outpouring of support and care from complete strangers made me feel like this was the right time for challenging the status quo.

If history is any indication, great movements and shifts in culture have started with one person having an idea. Take Rosa Parks in segregated America as an example. Her one act of defiance in refusing to obey the bus driver's order that she give up her seat in the coloured section to a white passenger, was the catalyst for human rights change across the entire country.

The other reason I feel so compelled to take this 'all the way' is because I know people want it. As individuals we will be forced to endure but collectively we have the power. While I might not have financial power to assist my cause, I have something even more powerful – people.

Who inspires you?

People like Denise and Bruce Morcombe, parents of Daniel who was murdered here in Australia a few years ago. They have turned their heartbreak and sorrow into a program for keeping kids safe. They now tirelessly spend their days educating and sharing their story to ensure no child has to go through what Daniel did, and no parent has to suffer the pain of losing a child. Such selfless people, doing extraordinary things for people everywhere.

Generally speaking I adore and admire people that despite great odds and adversity are able to get up and push through. And of course people who think about others more than they think about themselves.

Muktar Mai, a Pakistani woman from the village of Meerwala, is someone else that inspires me. I first heard about her when I read the book *Half the Sky* by Nicholas D Kristof and Sheryl WuDunn. Basically Muktar's story goes like this:

In July 2002 Muktar was gang raped by a group of men, on the orders of the council of a powerful clan, in revenge for a supposed sexual indiscretion by her younger brother. She was then forced to walk home, half naked, through a heckling crowd.

Feelings of fear and shame associated with being raped often stops the victim contacting the police, therefore most assaults go unreported. A lot of Pakistani women commit suicide because they can't bear the perceived disgrace and dishonour of being raped. But Muktar did something different. She went to the police and insisted that the accused were arrested, and then she went on to successfully challenge her attackers in court and won. The men were jailed.

This entire story up until now is inspirational, but what she did next really demonstrates the depth of this woman's courage. Using the money that she was given for compensation, Muktar opened up a school for the girls of her village. She wanted to inspire hope for their future through education and empowerment.

Muktar has become a symbol of hope for voiceless and oppressed women. She is a woman I admire greatly. There are many women like Muktar around the world. Inspiration is out there, if people used the right currency to look for it, they would see it everywhere.

CHAPTER TWENTY TWO

Where to from here?

IF YOU HAD TOLD ME FIVE YEARS AGO that I would be here, feeling the way I feel and doing what I do, I would've pushed you over Elaine Benes style from *Seinfeld* and said, 'Get out!' Never in my wildest dreams did I anticipate being so revealing to the world, including sharing nude photos and intimate stories.

It is hard to connect with the person I was just a few short years ago when I was standing in front of the mirror pulling my belly and telling myself that I was hideous. It makes me really sad to think of that dark place, but it also makes me feel inspired too. Inspired because I know that if I can make changes to improve my self-esteem, and go from hating to loving my body, then it's possible for many others to do the same. I'm inspired by the life that I live now and it's a life I want to encourage millions of others to have too. The reason I wrote this book was to share that message.

This wasn't part of any grand plan. I didn't wake up one day and say to myself, 'I am going to attempt to create global change.' Or, 'I am going to lead a movement that will change people's lives.' I mean who does that anyway? The road I've taken hasn't been strategically planned in advanced, but instead grew in the most organic, transparent and authentic way I've ever seen.

My drive and inspiration comes from YOU. I've been so humbled by the love and support I've received from strangers all over the world. I've spent more time in awe in the past couple of years than I have been in my life. I've always known that I was here for a purpose to help, it has always been what has fed my soul and now that my purpose has been unveiled I can't help but feel an incredible sense of freedom, to be doing what I am meant to do. This brings a feeling of responsibility. There is so much to be done, so much change to create, so many people to connect with, so many places to go. The unusual and exciting part of the responsibility, though, is that I don't feel fearful or intimidated, I feel motivated, driven, and most of all ready.

So many times in the past two years I've wondered why certain things in my life happened, and questioned why other things didn't. But now I understand the hurdles, the triumphs, the rejections, the mistakes, the lessons, the wins and the losses. They are all life experiences, valuable for different reasons, I get that now and it feels amazing.

I feel that Jason's death brought me and Mat together, and despite our rocky moments together, we were meant to share our lives. He moderates my wildest and most crazy ideas, we balance each other perfectly.

I think that being bullied at school gave me empathy for others.

Even though I met Kelley during a really difficult time she became one of the most important people in my life, and has provided me with strength, courage and wisdom.

Learning to be photographer was a great investment, because it gave me the skills I've needed for making a documentary, and it also delivered me a bunch of beautiful friends.

Taking part in the bodybuilding competition taught me how to love my body 'after' and made the 'before and after' photo possible.

I am blessed with the most hands-on, loving, caring, supportive and generous parents. Without them I wouldn't be standing.

Messing up that big presentation in Singapore taught me to never sit on the sidelines again.

Joining a mothers group against my better judgement when Oliver was a baby, meant I got to meet Emma Johnston, who has provided me with endless support, wise words and encouragement.

Deciding to video my Developing Daughters, Supporting Sons seminar meant that I met Hugh Fenton.

Having Mikaela helped me realise how important it is that we think about what kind of world our daughters are going to inherit.

All roads have led me here and coincidence has played no part, everything that has happened has happened for a reason and it feels amazing.

So where to from here? Well the road is long and it's definitely not paved smooth but I am ready for the challenge. By holding seminars, writing this book, filming the documentary, running local school programs and body image workshops and continuing to petition and campaign I hope to achieve the following:

I want people to change the currency of beauty from appearance to unseen qualities.

I want girls and boys to grow up respecting and loving their bodies.

I want more humans to buck trends, break rules and stand up for what they believe in.

I want people to value their health more than their beauty.

I want people to focus less on what they want and more on what others need.

I want people to learn perspective so they can live with more gratitude in their life.

I want people to see the beauty in humility, kindness and compassion and not in thigh gaps, flat stomachs and toned arms.

I want people who are in positions of power to flex their muscles for the good of humanity and not for record profits.

And from a less philosophical perspective...

I never want to hear:

'I don't like having my photo taken.'

'I am on a diet.'

'Does my bum look big in this?'

'I wish I had her boobs.'

'I hate my body.'

'Have you lost weight?'

Right now I am happy, content and more than anything equipped and prepared to take on the challenge of creating global change.

Life is really busy with the three kids, and I do have a lot of balls in the air. I have just released UNSTOPPABLE – an online program to help women to reach their potential, we are filming the documentary *Embrace* and in between that I am throwing kicks at karate, coaching the Under 8s soccer team and strumming a guitar quite badly. I am optimistic about a future in which I see myself traveling around the world, speaking and sharing my stories and stories of other women I have met on this journey of life. My favourite thing to do is to connect with people and I've discovered that I am quite a hugger, I love to hug everyone that believes in me, supports the movement, and champions my message. The movement is one big family of people working together to create positive change.

And if I'm right in assuming that you want to live in a world similar to the one I do, then you need to stand up and make a difference with me. You can by supporting me on social media:

Join the Body Image Movement.

If you go to www.bodyimagemovement.com.au there is a yellow sign up box. All you need to do is pop your email in there, that's it! It is a great way for us to stay connected and if I have something important to communicate with you, I can.

Follow Body Image Movement on Social Media.

Facebook: Body Image Movement

Twitter:

Taryn: @tarynbrumfitt

BIM: @bodyimagemvmt

Instagram: BODYIMAGEMOVEMENT

Use the hashtag #ihaveembraced on social media

I encourage you to share posts on social media, it really helps to get the message out and don't forget to tell all your friends about Body Image Movement!

And finally above all else I want you to believe:

Believe in yourself.

Believe that you can love your body.

and

Believe that together we can create positive global change.

 So the time has come for us to say goodbye. I sincerely thank you for allowing me to be part of your life and please remember: 'your body is not an ornament, it is the vehicle to your dreams.' x

ACKNOWLEDGEMENTS

Thanks to:

My tribe, Mathew, Oliver, Cruz and Mikaela, you guys are the bomb! I couldn't adore you anymore than I do, as I often say to you: 'I love you so much I think my heart is going to burst!' Thanks for your endless understanding and encouragement, and for being with me every step of the way.

Special mention to Mat, your role in all this has not been easy! When times were tough, you pushed through with me, you've been my endless sounding board, you've put up with my flighty moods and given the movement everything it needed. Thanks.

My mum and dad for providing me with everything I ever needed. Thanks for your endless support, love, generosity and kindness, you've given me a lifetime of treasured memories. I couldn't ask for better parents. Dad I am grateful for your wise words, and Mum your overabundance of selfless acts that have made my life a little less chaotic! (You know what I am talking about!)

Emma Johnston for your wise words and your unique ability to transform complicated long-winded strategies into practical and digestible plans of attack. And most importantly for being a great travel companion, thanks for keeping me calm on flights, and not being too high maintenance for twin bed arrangements!

Heath Vogt, I thank you for your endless flexibility, your patience, and for taking all my calls when something goes wrong or something goes right! Twelve months ago I promised you I would be less 'reactive' and more 'proactive' so we weren't always chasing our tail. I promise that time is coming!

Kate Ellis for taking the infamous Before and After photographs! Along with all my beautiful photography friends for having my back. It wasn't easy leaving my photography circle, especially since we had all just found each other, it is so comforting to know that our friendship goes beyond the camera.

School mums! Kim, Emma, Fiona, Kellie and Danielle. Thanks so much for being part of the 'roster' when I travel, and for being more than just school mums friends. Friends for life regardless of whether our kids are, I love you all.

Ellen de Generes. Just thanking you in advance, Ellen, I am sure by the time this book hits the shelves, your people would've spoken to my people and the magic will be in the pipeline!

Jason Butterworth, Aunty Ronda, Kelley McPhee, Steven McArthur, Nigel Marsh, Bec Derrington, Rachel Wade, Hugh Fenton, Operation Global Change, New Holland Publishers and all the friends that believed in me, supported me and loved me.

ABOUT THE AUTHOR

A lover of life, people and most of all, her husband and three children, Taryn Brumfitt is the founder and infectious voice behind the Body Image Movement - a global movement to shift the way women think about themselves, and in turn, feel about their bodies.

Writer, speaker and free spirit, Taryn is an internationally recognised positive body image activist rubbing shoulders with the likes of Beyoncé and Kate Moss in *Brigette* magazine's acclaimed 'Women of The Year' awards and with her powerful message reaching over 100 million people worldwide via social media.

A keynote speaker and presenter, Taryn is most passionate about creating a generation of empowered women through delivering her seminar Developing Daughters and Supporting Sons and her online program Unstoppable.

Interviewed by *Good Morning America*, *60 Minutes* and *The Today Show* and featured on the cover of *Women's Health and Fitness*, Taryn's latest project, Embrace the documentary, has been supported by the likes of Rosie O'Donnell, Zooey Deschanel, Ashton Kutcher and Ricki Lake after a whopping 9 million viewers were moved by its compelling trailer.

She enjoys dancing like no one is watching (even when people are), sipping on green smoothies, kicking butt at karate and reading books in a hammock...oh, and famously rockin' a pair of pink and orange glasses!